SUGAR ADDICTS' DIET

See the Pounds Drop Off!

By the same author:

Nicki Waterman's Flat Stomach Plan

SUGAR ADDICTS' DIET

See the Pounds Drop Off!

Nicki Waterman

and

MARTHA ROBERTS

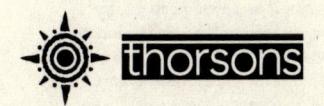

thorsons

Thorsons
An Imprint of HarperCollins*Publishers*
77–85 Fulham Palace Road,
Hammersmith
London W6 8JB

The website address is: www.thorsonselement.com

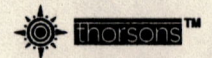

thorsons™

and *Thorsons* are trademarks of
HarperCollins*Publishers* Ltd

Published by Thorsons 2004

© Nicki Waterman 2004

Nicki Waterman asserts the moral right to
be identified as the author of this work

A catalogue record of this book
is available from the British Library

ISBN 978-0-00-732367-8

All rights reserved. No part of this publication may be
reproduced, stored in a retrieval system, or transmitted,
in any form or by any means, electronic, mechanical,
photocopying, recording or otherwise, without the prior
permission of the publishers.

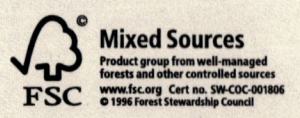

Mixed Sources
Product group from well-managed
forests and other controlled sources
www.fsc.org Cert no. SW-COC-001806
© 1996 Forest Stewardship Council

FSC is a non-profit international organisation established to
promote the responsible management of the world's forests.
Products carrying the FSC label are independently certified
to assure consumers that they come from forests that are
managed to meet the social, economic and ecological needs
of present and future generations.

Find out more about HarperCollins and the environment at
www.harpercollins.co.uk/green

Contents

Acknowledgements vii
Introduction: Nicki's Story 1

Part 1: The Truth about Sugar Addiction 9
1. Are You a Sugar Addict? 11
2. How This Book Can Help 29
3. Why We Crave Sugar 35
4. Why Do I Need to Break My Addiction? 57
5. Young Sugar Addicts 77
6. Helping Young Sugar Addicts 93
7. Where Sugar is Lurking 113

Part 2: The Sugar Addict's Tools for Recovery 117
8. What to Eat 119
9. How to Eat 145
10. Kick Out Sugar with Exercise 165
11. Hints and Tips for Giving Up 191
12. Coping with Sugar 'Dealers' 201

Part 3: Break Your Sugar Addiction in Three Weeks 233

13 The 21-day Plan   235
14 Menu Plans   285
15 Recipes to Help You Give Up Sugar   295

Afterword: What Next?   333
Bibliography   335
Useful Organizations   337

Acknowledgements

Nicki Waterman:
With thanks to: Amanda Ursell; Tania Alexander; Nick Canham; Sheila; Alfie; Jane; my brothers and sisters-in-law Freddy and Helen and Colin and Laura; my husband Dennis and children Alexandra and Harry. Without their help and support this book would never have been written.

Martha Roberts:
Dr Sarah Schenker, Professor Marie Reid, Dr Paul Chadwick, Dr Neal Barnard, Professor Aubrey Sheiham, Sue Keane, Stephen Lawson (Linus Pauling Institute), Trudi Gilmore, my husband Simon.

Introduction: Nicki's Story

As a fitness expert, I am regularly told, 'You're so lucky that you're so slim.' I always think, 'You don't know the half of it!' I may be slim now, but that hasn't always been the case. And even though I work hard to be this way, I used to fight a personal demon every minute of the day – my desire to eat sugar.

It was sugar that made me a chubby child and a chunky teenager. And in my 20s I gained even more weight thanks to my sweet tooth. Two pregnancies in quick succession made my weight problem even worse. My husband (now my ex) loved my spare tyres and discouraged my attempts to lose weight. I tried every diet under the sun, had acupuncture and hypnotherapy, and even resorted to slimming pills to shift the weight. But it didn't go – in fact, it all came back on and more.

DISCOVERING EXERCISE

My saving grace, 18 years ago, was discovering the importance of exercise. An inspirational trainer got me off the powerful prescription drugs I'd grown dependent on. As a result, I lost five stone and decided to spread the word about how weight loss could really improve your life.

But behind the scenes I had developed an unhealthy tactic to keep slim. I'd learned that by exercising in excess, I could still eat the sweets I wanted and maintain a reasonable weight. I'd developed my own eating pattern – one proper meal a day and plenty of sugary foods – to sustain this weight loss. I knew it wasn't healthy but it worked. Maintaining my weight loss, however, was a constant struggle. Although I looked slim, I was still flabby and covered in fat, despite my exercise regime. **I was a 'slim, fat person' – someone with the unhealthy attitudes of an overweight person contained within a slim frame.**

SHOCK DISCOVERY

I could have carried on like this for ever. I looked fine and no one would ever have known about my secret eating habits. But just a year ago, something shocked me into realizing that I had to change my ways. My mother-in-law was in hospital being treated for cancer. One day, when I was visiting her, her specialist came to talk to us about what she should eat when she came out of hospital. I'll never forget his words – 'Do not touch refined sugars – they will kill you.'

Thinking about how much sugar I was consuming on a daily basis made me realize that it could easily be me lying on my deathbed if I didn't drastically mend my ways. **On an average day I'd happily consume at least half a pound of pick 'n' mix (my big weakness), large**

Introduction

packets of American hard gums and jelly beans, a packet of biscuits and anything else that came my way (I can't believe I'm admitting this to you!). Putting an end to my sugar addiction wasn't just about me but other people too. I had a responsibility to my two children, husband, brothers and friends. This was the wake-up call I needed to help me tackle my serious sugar addiction head-on. I told all my friends, family and work colleagues that I needed their help and support. I was giving up sugar completely, and that meant no chocolate, biscuits, cakes – or pick 'n' mix.

GETTING STARTED

Like all addicts, my decision to kick my habit wasn't without pain – I endured three weeks of excruciating headaches, something I found almost unbearable but knew I had to go through. Different addicts have their own preferred method for distracting themselves in moments of weakness. A nicotine addict might chew a pen as a substitute for having a cigarette in their mouth. I knew I needed something to stop me going into the local newsagent to get my sugar kick, so I starting boxing lessons with a professional coach. While I was focusing on boxing, I wasn't yearning for my next sugar fix.

Every time I ate something, I'd text my best friend so we had a record. I didn't trust myself to write it down honestly. Different people – including friend and nutritionist Amanda Ursell – advised me on what to eat to help get me through my cravings.

DEVISING THE SUGAR ADDICTS' DIET

But before I knew it, I was falling off the wagon. Willpower and exercise alone weren't enough. I soon realized there was no point in just giving up sugar unless my diet was right too. Looking into it, I began to understand that I needed support – both physical and emotional – if my attempts to give up sugar were to succeed. That's when I decided to devise my own sugar addicts' diet. **My aim was to even out my blood sugar levels, which I was told were probably a key part of my cravings. This would ensure I was never hungry (so never tempted by sugar!) and make me more capable of dealing with the inevitable emotions of trying to kick the sugar habit.** To be honest, at first I was a little sceptical that it would make a difference to my life. However, I can honestly say – hand on heart – that the 21-day plan really did work for me.

The weight has fallen off me and so has the body fat. I have achieved this without the need for over-exercising, which is just as bad for your body as doing no exercise at all. It's hard for me to believe that I don't have a weight problem for the first time in my life.

Introduction

A HEALTH-BOOSTING DIET PLAN

The Sugar Addicts' Diet has had countless benefits besides reducing my weight and body fat. I used to wake up with big dark rings under my eyes, and my skin had an unhealthy pallor. I put it down to ageing but, since kicking the sugar habit, I realize my diet was to blame. In my experience, the old saying 'You are what you eat' is so true. The bags under my eyes have now gone, my eyes look bright, my skin glows with health and my hair is thicker. The sugar highs and lows are a thing of the past, which means I have so much more energy than ever before.

I'm not saying I don't ever have cravings, but I seem to be able to control them a lot better. I control them – they don't control me, as they did in the past. A big part of it has been developing strategies to help me avoid situations in which I might be tempted to slip off the straight and narrow.

A WIDESPREAD ADDICTION

Since I made the decision to tackle my sugar addiction, I've discovered how many 'secret' addicts there are out there. 'And I thought I was the only one like that!' is something I now hear a lot. **Sugar is everywhere and it's hard to avoid it. That's why it can be such a battle to kick your addiction. But I've come a long way, and I want other people to know they can do it too. Like me, you will find you lose excess weight, feel**

fantastic – and lay the foundations for a longer and healthier life.

I've been shocked by people's lack of knowledge about the hidden sugars in their diet. There are confusing messages about sugar all around us, whether it's on food labels or in fast-food joints. I have written this book to help sugar addicts like me understand why they crave sugar, and how they can get it out of their system and beat the craving once and for all.

A HEALTHY EATING PROGRAMME FOR LIFE

My co-author, Martha Roberts, is an experienced, award-winning health writer with an avid interest in nutrition. She's also one of the few people I know who isn't addicted to sugar.

People often say if you want something done, ask a busy person. Well, it could also be said that if you want to understand how to enjoy non-sugary food, ask a person who's not hooked on it! Together, as a writing team, we represent two opposite sides of the sugar-eating spectrum. We hope to present an unbiased, balanced view of how sugar affects all of our lives.

The Sugar Addicts' Diet is a healthy eating programme for life. It will teach you about sugar so that you understand what it does for you (both good and bad), where it is in your food and how you can have more control over it so that it no longer controls you.

Introduction

It's really about lifestyle – learning skills for life and changing your ways without too much effort or heartache. And whether you're reading this book because you want to lose weight or you're fed up with being controlled by sugar, we hope it gives you the guidance and support you need to finally kick your sugar habit for good.

Part 1:

The Truth about Sugar Addiction

1
Are You a Sugar Addict?

For many of us, being told how something can affect our health in the future is a big yawn. We're told smoking can kill us and the sun can age us. Now we're being told that sugar is one of our biggest enemies. It seems everyone's out to get us. But many of us have the philosophy, 'Why deprive yourself now on the off-chance that you will get ill in years to come?'

While eating sugar might not send you to the grave, it can lead to problems such as obesity and related illnesses that can make your life a misery. **Symptoms or conditions linked to eating too much sugar may not be life-threatening but they can certainly threaten your quality of life.** Even the government is now worried about the amount of sugar in our diets and has pledged to put it on its health 'hit list' after salt. And even before you start to suffer from the types of medical condition outlined in Chapter 4, chances are you're already suffering from sugar overload. This can lead to troublesome symptoms that spoil your sense of health and wellbeing.

OUR NATURAL LOVE OF SUGAR

Most of us love sugar. We are biologically driven to enjoy sweetness because it helps us identify foods that are safe to eat rather than poisonous (as bitter foods might suggest). Experiments on 10-day-old babies show that when an adult gives them a dummy dipped in sugar solution, they gurgle and look pleased when they see that adult again. Our desire for sweetness is something we can learn from a very young age – and never forget.

But an extreme love of sugar isn't an inevitability – that's something we can prompt by our actions when selecting foods for our children. Professor Aubrey Sheiham, Professor of Dental Public Health at University College London, has written extensively on sugars and health. He says there's a crucial 'window' for overdeveloping this natural preference for sweetness in children and it becomes apparent when a child is weaning. At this point, they become 'picky' as they learn which foods are likely to be 'safe' and which are likely to be 'harmful'. If this preference is indulged with lots of highly sweet foods, they will generally prefer sweet foods from that point onwards. Professor Sheiham says, 'If you give them lots of sweet food in that window between the ages of two and four, their threshold and their liking for sugar will increase and they'll want more. Equally, if you give them mildly sweet things, like fruit, their threshold will be lower.'

Are You a Sugar Addict?

So what can you do if you're an adult with a sweet tooth? It is possible to retrain your sweet tooth so that you lower your sweetness threshold. One former sugar addict, Amila, says, 'My love of chocolate meant that nothing but chocolate could satisfy my sugar cravings. But I've now weaned myself off it by eating other sweet foods such as fruit, and where I used to eat bars of chocolate at a time to get the sweetness I needed, I now find that just one piece of chocolate is sweet enough for me. It really has been a case of "retraining" my palate. If you'd told me before that you could do this, I'd never have believed you!' As you'll see as you read through this book, stabilizing your blood-sugar levels through a proper diet, and finding sweetness in new places such as fruit, can help you retrain your own palate. This also has implications for preventing your children from loving sugar too much (see Chapters 5 and 6).

WHAT IS SUGAR ADDICTION?

If you simply love sugar, does it mean you have a sugar addiction? Doesn't it just mean you really enjoy the sugar taste and experience? It's when enjoyment turns to compulsion – a need – that we begin to get into the realms of addiction. An addiction is:

- an intense desire for a substance, a desire so severe it disrupts normal life
- very difficult to stop

- something that prompts a severe physiological (bodily) response upon stopping.

People who are addicted to something experience a loss of control over their behaviour. They use a substance repetitively and compulsively, despite knowing it might have undesirable consequences. Some experts say that, unlike cigarettes, alcohol and other drugs, there is still insufficient scientific proof that physical addiction to sugar truly exists.

But many people say that their own overwhelming desire to eat sugar is proof enough. Some studies have also suggested that addiction to sugar can be demonstrated. In 2002, a psychologist at Princeton University showed in experiments that rats not only eat sugar excessively, but they suffer from withdrawal when denied it and continue to crave it weeks later. However, as we'll see in Chapter 2, other experts suggest our desire for sugar (or, as they suggest, sugary, fatty foods) is more emotional than physical.

Whatever it is, there are lots of you out there who can't get through the day without thinking about sugar – and probably eating it in excess, too. We don't claim to be able to sort out the emotional side of why you want to eat sugar. That may be based on years of learning and habit, and addressing it may require soul-searching and even professional help. However, by focusing on sugar 'dealers' in Chapter 12, we hope to help you see that there could be emotional trigger points to your desire for sugar. In combination with our 21-day plan, this will help you start to feel on a more even keel, physically and emotionally, when it comes to your desire to eat sugar.

> ### Nicki's Personal Addiction
>
> *My sugar addiction was with me all the time. Sugar was an obsession – the desire for it, how I was going to get it and how long it would be before I could taste it. I just wasn't satisfied until I knew I could have that fix. Even a five-course meal wouldn't satisfy the yearning for sugar. It's as if there was a 'good' voice and a 'bad' voice inside my head. The good voice told me, 'You shouldn't be eating the sugar and should choose something else instead'. The bad voice said, 'Go on – go for it! You know you want to…' I felt out of control, as if sugar had cast a spell on me and I was powerless to do anything against it.*

What Other People Say about their Sugar Addiction

As soon as we told people we were writing a book about sugar addiction, they said, 'That's ME!' *Everyone* we mentioned it to said they had a problem with sugar cravings. Before we started out, we thought we'd strike a chord but we didn't realize it would be to this extent.

SUGAR ADDICTS' DIET

Here are some of the things they say about their love of sugar:

'I have to have it in the house or I don't feel secure.'

'Even after a huge meal I have to have two sweets to be truly satisfied.'

'I've loved sugar ever since I was a child.'

'I'll ask to see the dessert menu before I order anything else – I often build the entire meal around the dessert.'

'If I eat too much sugar I feel drained of energy, I struggle to open my eyes and I sleep more.'

'Too much sugar and I feel like I have a hangover.'

Are You a Sugar Addict?

> ### Polly's Story
>
> *I've been hooked on sugar since childhood. Sugar is a device I use to make me feel happy. But as well as giving me pleasure, I abuse it. Some days I really try and get myself in check. I think, 'How can I let sugar rule my life?' But it's so powerful I sometimes feel it's no different to someone who is on heroin.*

Sugar Addiction: the Symptoms

Losing control over your behaviour when sugar is around, eating it repetitively and compulsively, problems stopping its use – already this may sound familiar to you. But to give you further guidance, listed below are physical and emotional symptoms experienced by many people who say they can't live without sugar. As we'll see in later chapters, addiction is often linked to the emotions sugar stirs up in you. But it's also about what it does to you physically.

The symptoms listed here are typical of imbalances in blood sugar levels. They also reflect a diet low in nutrients and high in sugars and refined carbohydrates. Poor eating habits, such as not eating regularly enough, make matters worse. The Sugar Addicts' Diet addresses all these imbalances to help reduce such symptoms.

As you read through these lists, you may recognize

some – or even all – of these symptoms. However, even people who have none of these symptoms will find the Sugar Addicts' Diet a sensible, healthy, balanced eating plan that will help them maintain good health and prevent these symptoms taking hold.

Physical Symptoms
- Trouble controlling your weight
- Restlessness followed by a slump
- Lack of energy
- Trouble concentrating
- Dizziness and/or visual disturbances
- Headaches
- Tiredness and drowsiness, especially during the day
- Insomnia
- Cravings
- PMS
- Any of the conditions defined in Chapter 4

Emotional Symptoms
- Irritable and easily stressed
- Frustration and anxiety
- Mood swings
- Miserable, even tearful
- Nervousness
- Never feeling fully satisfied with food
- Euphoria when you first eat sugar

Are You a Sugar Addict?

- Lying about how much sugar you eat
- Taking extreme measures to get sugar (e.g. midnight visit to the shops)
- Confusion about what to do to feel better

You may well have gone through the lists saying, 'That's me!' To confirm that you have a problem with sugar, take a look at the checklist below. Some people who crave sugar, like Nicki, describe the following:

Checklist: Are You a Sugar Addict?
Answer 'yes' or 'no' to the following statements:

- **You think about sugary foods more than any other types of food. YES/NO**

Nicki says, 'Every minute of the day, from the moment I woke up to the moment I went to bed, I'd think about sweet food, whether it was sweets, chocolate, biscuits or cakes. I'd even wake in the middle of the night thinking of it.'

- **You've attempted to cut down on sweet food in your diet before. YES/NO**

Nicki says, 'I've lost count of the number of times I've said, "Right, that's it – from today I'm giving up sugary foods" and succeeded for a couple of days, only to be drawn back in by blinding headaches, grumpiness and sheer desire for sugar.'

SUGAR ADDICTS' DIET

- **You find yourself eating more and more sugar as time goes by. YES/NO**

Nicki says, 'I ate a lot of sugar as a child and somehow managed to kid myself that I didn't eat as much as an adult, but I definitely did. Back then it was a treat – as an adult you can make it part of your everyday life and no one will question you.'

- **You lie about how much sugary food you eat. YES/NO**

Nicki says, 'I've lied so many times to friends, family and colleagues about how much sugar I've eaten. There's direct lying, like "I haven't eaten any sugar today" when I have, and indirect lying where I haven't corrected people when they assume I never waver from a healthy diet.'

- **If you miss out on regular sugar, you feel terrible. YES/NO**

Nicki says, 'If I didn't eat sugar regularly enough, I was like a monster – irritable, grumpy, headachy and unable to sit still. It was as if I'd been possessed and the only thing that would put it right was a sugar fix.'

- **You've altered your routine to get sweet foods. YES/NO**

Nicki says, 'When I needed sugar and didn't have the right foods in the house, I'd make special arrangements to get it, whether it was leaving home half an hour early to ensure I could stop for it or ringing friends and asking them to pick it up on the way to see me.'

Are You a Sugar Addict?

- **The thought of getting sugar makes you focused and tunnel-visioned. YES/NO**

Nicki says, 'I know all the newsagents near me that sell pick 'n' mix – and I used to use them as landmarks. If I knew I was going near one and had the opportunity for a "fix", it was as if my senses were on red alert and my concentration was at its peak.'

- **You've experienced what feels like a sugar 'hangover'. YES/NO**

Nicki says, 'I've had some memorable alcohol hangovers in my time but my worst hangovers have definitely been after sugar binges. I felt nauseous, headachy and struggled to get out of bed.'

- **You often feel sugar is ruling you. YES/NO**

Nicki says, 'Anyone who doesn't have a thing about sugar probably thinks it's strange to say this, but it really can feel as though sugar is controlling your life, from your hunger levels and taste buds through to your emotions. My idea of freedom is being able to say "no" to sugar without a second thought.'

- **You often binge on sweet foods or white-flour foods such as biscuits or cakes. YES/NO**

Nicki says, 'I've lost count of the number of times I've binged on biscuits, freshly toasted white bread, pick 'n' mix or cakes. When you love sugar, it becomes an intrinsic part of your life.'

If you've said 'yes' to two or more of these, you have a problem with sugar. Don't worry – we're going to try and help you. Even if this isn't you, this book will still be of interest, not least in helping you to understand the behaviour of others around you – perhaps friends or relatives who struggle with weight issues or ill health and don't even realize that sugar could be to blame.

SUGAR IS EVERYWHERE

Picture it – you wake up in the morning and have a bowl of cereal and a cup of tea. You'll already have eaten more than 8 grams of sugar if you've had a bowl of cornflakes – make that 44 grams if it's a bowl of Frosties. And that's before you've sprinkled sugar on top of your cereal and put two spoons of it in your tea.

As a nation we're eating more sugar than ever before. The average Briton eats 16 times more sugar today than 100 years ago. In 1900, people ate an average of 4 pounds (around 1.5 kilos) of sugar a year – the equivalent of around a bag and a half of sugar. Today, according to the UK's National Diet and Nutrition Survey, that figure is 65 pounds or just over 24 kilos – the equivalent of 24 bags of sugar every year. That's around 65 grams – 13 teaspoons – a day. In the US, added sugar can comprise as much as a quarter of a person's daily food intake.

You might think, 'But I don't even buy that many bags of sugar in a year.' True, you probably don't. That's because the figure comes not just from the sugar we actively put in our food, by sprinkling it on cereal or spooning it into tea and coffee. It also includes the 'hidden' sugar that's so often put into our food at the manufacturing stage, and which we may not even understand we're consuming. Food manufacturers are being increasingly pressurized by parents, campaign groups, politicians and health experts to reduce levels of sugar, fat and salt in certain foods and to call a halt to advertising foods to children (an issue we look into in Chapter 5). The Food and Drink Federation, which represents food manufacturers, announced that supersize chocolate snacks are due to be axed to help in the battle against obesity, which is a step in the right direction. But in the meantime, the onus is on us to be vigilant and look out for sugar for ourselves.

How Much Sugar Should We Eat?
The UK government and the World Health Organization recommend that starchy carbohydrates such as bread, rice and pasta should constitute 55–75 per cent of our daily food intake. Free sugars or 'non-milk extrinsic sugars' – sugar added by us or, more significantly, by the manufacturer – should comprise 10 per cent or less. In other words, no more than one-tenth of our daily calories should come from added sugar.

If the average woman's recommended daily calorie intake is 1,940 (less if you are overweight and want to shift some pounds), that means no more than 194 calories should come from added sugar. But, as we have seen, the average Briton is already on 65 grams, or a huge 260 calories, of these added sugars per day, 30 per cent more than the recommended maximum. A can of cola contains just over 10 teaspoons of sugar (200 calories) so you can see how easy it is to go over the advised amount. Have a think about how many cans of soft drink, biscuits, cakes, sweets and bowls of cereal you eat in any one day and you'll probably find this is way more than one-tenth of the food you eat, and far in excess of 10 teaspoons of sugar.

> ### Nicki's Tip
>
> *Want to work out how much sugar there is in a food? Take a look at the label. Where it says 'carbohydrates', it generally says 'of which sugars – Xg'. A teaspoon of sugar is around 5g so divide X by 5 to find out how many teaspoons of sugar it contains. So if it says 'of which sugars – 15g', divide 15 by 5 and you'll know it contains 3 teaspoons.*

Are You a Sugar Addict?

THE SUGAR CONTENT OF FOODS

Food	Rounded Teaspoons of Extrinsic (Added) Sugar
1 digestive biscuit	½
1 chocolate digestive	1
1 slice (45g) of jam-filled sponge cake	4
Mars Bar	7
1 milk chocolate bar (50g)	5½
1 scoop of ice cream	1½
1 bowl of cornflakes	½
1 teaspoon of jam	¾
Half a tin (200ml) of cream of tomato soup	1
Half a tin of baked beans	2½
1 glass of Lucozade	6
1 glass of Ribena	4
1 tablespoon of tomato ketchup	1
1 tablespoon of sweet pickle	1
1 tablespoon of salad cream	½
1 can (300ml) of cola	7

Where Sugar is 'Hiding'

Even people whose diet consists mainly of savoury rather than sweet foods are probably eating more sugar than they realize, especially if they are fans of processed foods such as ready meals. **The last thing you expect to find in a savoury ready meal is sugar, right? Wrong! They can contain up to 20 per cent sugar.** And what about the sugar found in a dollop of tomato ketchup? Remember: even so-called 'low-fat' foods can be high in sugar.

The problem is that sugar is often added to foods where you'd never expect to find it. Would you, in a million years, ever imagine that there's sugar in some sandwich meats or certain varieties of cottage cheese? For further jaw-dropping revelations about where you're likely to find sugar when you least expect it, see Chapter 7.

If you really want to avoid sugar, you have to learn how to decipher labels and get to the root of what you're being fed. Sometimes it can feel like you're reading another language! In later chapters, we'll show you how to be a label 'detective' and work out for yourself if a food contains sugar, even if it looks like it shouldn't.

DOES OUR LOVE OF SUGAR REALLY MATTER?

Does it really matter that we're eating so much sugar? It tastes great and it makes us feel happy and content. Many of us would say there's no high that compares to the buzz of eating sugar. But the satisfaction comes at a price.

If you have a major love affair with sugar, chances are you're also having major problems with your weight. Later (see Chapter 3), we'll be explaining that sugar is a carbohydrate and that some carbohydrates in the diet are good. Chosen properly, they can actually help you maintain a steady weight and improve your health. We will also see that some sugars are preferable to others. But at the moment, all you need to know is that, by and large, sugar added to the diet is bad and is one of the main reasons we're now fatter than ever before.

As you'll see in Chapter 4, there is also a huge range of health problems that are either brought on or exacerbated by eating too much sugar. For every medical study that suggests sugar is good for you (and these are generally funded by the immensely powerful sugar industry), there are dozens more that warn of the negative impact of high-sugar diets that are now so familiar to us.

2
How This Book Can Help

So you're a sugar addict. Perhaps, after doing the questionnaire in Chapter 1, you've admitted this to yourself for the first time. That's an amazing first step – realizing you have an issue with sugar is a huge leap forward because it means you're now in a position to do something about it.

There are lots of self-help books about addiction, habits, cravings and, specifically, sugar. We should know – we've read them all. But we found most of them so difficult to read and understand that you could be forgiven for reaching for the sugar as a reward! This book intends to give you all this help and more in an uncomplicated way. The plan is based on Nicki's success at beating her sugar addiction, following her lifelong struggle with it. She says, 'When I decided to deal with my sugar addiction, I was faced with lots of conflicting messages about it – take this supplement, don't eat this, increase the amount of that. It was a nightmare. Having done it all and been through hell and back, I now feel I can share with you what works and what doesn't. You all know what sugar means to me, and if I can manage to kick the habit by following this plan, then so can you.'

OUR PHILOSOPHY

The aim of this book is to get you on the road to making the right food choices and eating regularly to help break the sugar habit *and* lose weight. Sounds simple, but so many of us with sugar addictions don't do this. By making these two things a habit, you can help to ensure you never feel that roaring hunger that so often accompanies diets. As a result, you should – like Nicki – start to feel more physically and emotionally balanced as your body responds to the good things you're feeding it and your need for sugar reduces. Stick with this and you'll eventually be at the stage where you can allow yourself a sugary treat (come on – we're all human!) and it won't draw you back into your old ways. Plus, you'll be losing weight *without* tedious calorie-counting. How's that for an incentive!

HOW THE DIET WORKS

We'll be going into a lot more detail about the right food choices, but here they are in a nutshell:

- **Avoid 'obvious' sugars and 'sneaky' sugars:** This will help prevent sugar 'highs and lows'.
- **Eat good-quality complex carbohydrates, protein and fibre together:** This will stop you

feeling hungry. Fibre (in complex carbohydrates or vegetables) helps to slow down the rate at which glucose is broken down in the body, thus helping to prevent sugar peaks and dips.
- **Include plenty of 'good' fats in the diet:** Omega 3 and 6 oils from fish, nuts and seeds boost carbohydrate metabolism, helping to burn carbohydrate calories more quickly.
- **Eat regularly and have good quality snacks:** Regular meals and snacking on the right foods will help to keep blood-sugar levels even through the day and prevent you bingeing.

The diet has worked a treat for many sugar addicts. Even those who didn't think they had poor blood-sugar control have found it's worked for them – this is an eating plan that can be used by just about anyone. As it's based on the principles of healthy eating and cutting out added sugars and refined carbohydrates, it's also suitable for diabetics. But if you have diabetes, always talk to your GP or specialist before changing your eating programme.

> ### Polly's Story
>
> *Before I sorted out my blood sugar, I'd get the shakes and would have to have sugar. If I got hungry, I'd lose the plot. By learning to eat properly – protein with carbohydrate – and have good, regular snacks, I've really helped to level things out. Now if I have sweet things, it's because I want them rather than need them, as I used to.*

How the Diet Can Help You

So how are we going to help you? What we aren't going to do is preach – there's nothing worse than some faceless person telling you what you can't eat or can't do. This is Nicki's story of how she got her sugar addiction under control and lost weight in the process – a true double-whammy! As you go through the book in your own efforts to get sugar back on your terms, Nicki will be with you all the way, giving you her tips, support and encouragement.

You probably don't associate the word 'diet' with fun, but we're going to show you that it doesn't necessarily have to mean 'punishment' either. By sorting out your relationship with sugar, you'll feel better physically and emotionally, not held to ransom by your love of it.

You're no doubt feeling bad about your love of sugar

How This Book Can Help

and won't want us to make you feel any worse. But early on we're going to tell you about how sugar can affect your health. First, because it's true, and second, because it could be the extra 'nudge' you need to make you address your problem once and for all. As you saw in the introduction, this is what happened to Nicki.

There may be times when you feel like giving up the diet. But before you do, remember this – Nicki was like you, wanting sugar all the time and feeling it controlled her life. She was also, believe it or not, carrying extra pounds that she couldn't shift. She managed to lose this extra weight simply by eating the Sugar Addicts' Diet way. She knows this is the formula for success, and she wants to share it with you.

Nicki's Tips

Throughout the book, Nicki will be offering her tips on how she kicked her sugar habit, from coping with those difficult 'no sugar' moments through to positive messages that have worked for her. Some might work for you, some might not – the important thing is to use these tips either as tools or simply inspiration to find your own methods for getting a grip on your sugar cravings. And if you find your own tips, tell us – we'd love to hear about them so we can pass them on.

What You Need

Keep a pen or pencil with you because you'll need it to write your diary. Keeping a food diary is a crucial part of the plan – there is a template in the book for you to copy and fill in yourself (as well as a version filled in by Nicki to show you how to do it).

You can record all kinds of information, from how sugar is making you feel and who your sugar 'dealers' are to the names of sugar-free foods you may hear someone mention on television. Don't worry – it won't be like going back to school! And believe us, it's not a waste of time. Nicki says, 'Being able to write things down was a vital part of my recovery programme. There's so much going on in your head when you're beating an addiction you really need that outlet. It also helps you to be true to yourself – it's so easy to lie about what you've been eating, but if you have to write it down, somehow it's different.'

3

Why We Crave Sugar

In the past, not a minute would go by without Nicki thinking about sugar. But why did she crave it? And why is it that you are so desperate for it? In Nicki's experience, her sugar addiction was made up of two parts – **physical** and **emotional**.

The physical was about the 'hit' and energy rush she got from sugar, while the emotional was about the role sugar played in terms of making her feel happy and comfortable. When she decided to tackle her addiction, she realized she was going to have to take a good look at both aspects if she was to succeed.

In helping you overcome your addiction in the same way, we can't just say to you, 'Stop eating sweets' or 'Chuck that chocolate in the bin'. That won't be the answer – it wasn't for Nicki. We need to explain to you what sugar is, where it is found in food and how it affects you physically. We'll also be looking at the emotional side of sugar, how it can be more than just a taste sensation but also a friend, comforter and reward. We explain that while the 'feel-good' factor from sugar is an emotion, there are physical factors to take into account, too, such as how sugar affects blood-sugar levels. In other words, **if you're hooked on sugar, it's not a case of 'lack of willpower'. There's a powerful combination of emotional and chemical activity inside you that's hard to beat!**

Bear with us through the explanation of what sugar is. It might sound complicated but it's crucial to your understanding of what it's doing when you eat it. It will also start to give you an insight into how you're going to beat it.

THE PHYSICAL ADDICTION
What is Sugar?
Sugar is what's known as a carbohydrate. Carbohydrates are fuel for the body and, as our bodies can't make them, we have to get them from our food. Compared to fats and protein, they are also the quickest-acting form of energy we can get.

The carbohydrates we eat come in two main varieties – simple and complex.

Simple Carbohydrates
These are what we most commonly refer to as sugars, or simple sugars. If you were to look at them under a microscope, you'd see that they are quite small, short units. Because of this, they are easily and quickly absorbed by the stomach or small intestine. You'll

recognize their scientific names because they end in '-ose', such as glucose and fructose.

Complex Carbohydrates
These are generally longer units – in fact, they are simple sugars strung together. Before they can be used by the body, they have to be broken down into smaller, simple units – a process that takes both time and energy.

In order to be used by the body, all carbohydrates are eventually broken down into glucose. We can see from this that glucose (a sugar) isn't *bad* – in fact, it's essential for life. The brain and nervous system need glucose to function. But we get the glucose we need from the breakdown of vegetables, fruits and grains without adding any extra. Also, if the production of glucose from the food is slow because the body has to break it down – as it does with 'brown', complex carbohydrates – this helps to regulate the amount of glucose in the blood. If, on the other hand, the breakdown is quick, this can lead to high amounts of glucose in the blood followed by a corresponding dip – poor blood-sugar control. And some carbohydrates cause this to happen more quickly than others. Simple carbohydrates get converted to glucose very quickly (if they aren't already glucose itself) while complex carbohydrates are absorbed into the bloodstream slowly, helping to avoid these blood-sugar imbalances. For further information about blood sugar, see 'The Sugar Roller Coaster', on page 39.

Stop! You're probably thinking that all complex carbohydrates must be good for you because your body has to work to break them down. That's not the case – some are far better than others. Complex carbohydrates come in two varieties – unrefined and refined.

UNREFINED CARBOHYDRATES
These are eaten pretty much as nature made them. Examples of unrefined complex carbohydrates are whole grains used in whole-grain bread, or brown rice complete with its husks. These release energy slowly in the body. With unrefined complex carbohydrates, the fibre – made up of glucose molecules strung together – cannot be broken down or digested, and as a result helps to slow down the speed at which the rest of the carbohydrate breaks down in the body.

REFINED CARBOHYDRATES
These are essentially 'sneaky' sugars that have been processed to extend their shelf-life and make them desirable to us shoppers. But in the process they've lost many of the nutrients that made them beneficial in the first place. These refined carbs are often lacking in essential minerals and vitamins. Importantly, they have also had their fibre – such as cellulose or pectin – taken away. It's this fibre that can help to slow down a carbohydrate's breakdown into glucose, which in turn helps to regulate blood-sugar levels. The fact that they

can be broken down so quickly after being eaten means these refined carbs are essentially just like simple sugars. But because so many of us don't know the effect they have on the body, they are hidden or 'sneaky' sugars.

As you'll see in Chapter 8, we'll be telling you about which foods you should eat to help stabilize blood sugar and minimize your sweet cravings. The carbohydrates we recommend are unrefined – refined carbs are a definite no-no.

The Sugar 'Roller Coaster'

When we eat simple or 'sneaky' sugars, they go straight into the blood. This huge 'hit' of sugar causes the body to flood the bloodstream with the sugar-control hormone, insulin, to try and regulate sugar levels. The trouble is that the body isn't designed for such high sugar levels – the most sugar our caveman ancestors would have got was from berries picked off bushes, not chocolate bars or jelly babies! Excessive amounts of insulin end up being released to deal with the sugar, either by removing it from the blood or taking it to the muscles.

Imagine a roller coaster which starts off at a low level, climbing to a high peak before dropping down into a dip. It's the same principle when you eat sugar. You start off with low amounts of sugar in the blood (the roller coaster dips), eat lots of sugar (the roller coaster rises), then insulin is produced to flush the excess sugar out, dropping sugar levels back down (the roller coaster dips again).

'So what?' you might think. Well, eating sugar – where the roller coaster peaks – and the rise in blood-sugar levels may make you feel high, happy and even euphoric. After all, that's one of the reasons sugar is so attractive. But the point at which the roller coaster falls – the 'sugar dip' – can leave you feeling tired, ratty and even depressed. As well as increasing your risk of certain illnesses (see Chapter 4) and putting on weight, it's this dip that can make you want to eat more sugar to get that roller coaster back on a high again. **If you don't break your sugar-eating habits, you're essentially destined for life on a sugar roller coaster that you're not allowed to get off.** Life on this roller coaster is a crucial part of sugar addiction.

Which Foods Fuel the Roller Coaster?

Simple sugars are perfect fuel for this blood-sugar roller coaster, as are the 'sneaky' sugars – the refined carbohydrates. The extent to which specific carbohydrates (including 'good' unrefined complex carbohydrates) make the roller coaster rise – and the speed at which they do so – depends on something called the Glycaemic Index (GI). The GI is a way of measuring the effects of food on blood-sugar levels. Foods range from high GI down to low GI.

High GI foods break down quickly during digestion and raise blood-sugar levels rapidly and to high levels. Examples include white rice (not basmati) and white bread.

Why We Crave Sugar

Mid GI foods break down moderately slowly. Examples include pasta and raisins.

Low GI foods break down slowly and release sugar gradually into the bloodstream for long-term energy. Examples include lentils, sweet potatoes, and fruits such as cherries and peaches.

In simple terms, if you want to stop the roller coaster – or at least stop it rising and falling so sharply – you should be trying to eat low GI foods rather than high GI ones. But don't start panicking and trying to work out what the GI rating of foods is. The Sugar Addicts' Diet incorporates these principles for you so foods we suggest you eat will tend to be low or medium GI, and those we advise cutting down on or removing altogether will tend to be high GI. We'll be providing you with lists of these foods later on, as well as a meal planner and recipes.

Nicki's Physical Addiction

'When I had a bag of sweets in front of me, I'd have that physical "rush" you get when something really exciting is about to happen to you. And when I ate them, they never disappointed. I'd get an intense, overwhelming rush of energy, taking me to a real high. I've never taken drugs but I often wonder if it's a similar feeling. The trouble was that I'd have to keep on eating the sweets to get that high feeling. In my world, there was no such thing as eating just one pink shrimp – I had to eat the lot. It was like being on a confectionery conveyor belt where the sweets kept coming and I kept eating. I never felt sick or reached "saturation point", which really added to the problem. If I'd felt ill, I might have been inclined to stop! But of course I had to stop eventually, not because willpower kicked in but because the sweets ran out and there was nothing more to binge on. When I saw the bottom of the bag, I'd feel really sad and deflated. After my sugar "high" it was like payback time – I'd have low energy and would start feeling weary. Other people picked up on it, too. They'd say, "What's the matter with you?"'

THE EMOTIONAL ADDICTION

As we've seen, a large part of sugar addiction is down to what sugar does when it gets into your body. Being on the sugar roller coaster means we feel terrible if we don't have sugar because of the dip that inevitably follows our sugar hit. Not surprisingly, many of us reach for sugar to lift us out of that trough and get us on a high again. However, the part that sugar plays in making us feel certain emotions such as happiness or relief is also central to addiction. Perhaps you were given sweets as a child as a reward for being good, or maybe you raided the kitchen cupboard for biscuits after being told off. Whatever it is, it's very likely you'll have associations with sugar that go back to when you were younger.

What the Experts Say
'It's more Emotional than Physical'
Marie Reid, Professor of Nutritional Psychology at the University of Surrey, Roehampton, has written widely on sugar addiction. She says studies have failed to prove that sugary foods lead to physiological addiction, such as you can get with alcohol or drugs. Rather, it's down to people making associations with certain feelings when they eat sugar. They may use it for comfort, for example, and if they're denied it they can start feeling miserable.

Professor Reid says, 'Research suggests that people are not addicted to sugar on a physical level but maybe on a psychological level. It comes from all the meaning we have around food – sugar is regarded as "forbidden" food. So if, from a very young age, there's an association with that kind of food as a treat, something used as reward or punishment, they take that all the way through their life. A familiar pattern would be that good behaviour was congratulated with something like chocolate so chocolate is seen as a reward food. Or they may have been given it when something went wrong, like they hurt themselves. That then moves into comfort eating to cheer themselves up when sad or miserable, or a reward when they feel happy, or both.'

The food used for these purposes could just as easily have been something healthy like fruit. But Professor Reid says, 'Sweet foods are often palatable, and humans have an innate preference for sweet foods – breast milk is sweet.' She suggests that the 'dependence-like addiction' people so often have isn't to sugar alone but rather to the combination of carbohydrates and fat – in other words, sugary, fatty foods such as cakes, chocolate and pastry. So as far as she's concerned, there's little evidence that an intense craving for sugar is down to anything physiological.

'It's Emotional AND Physical'

According to some experts, sugar acts on brain chemicals as well as having an effect on blood-sugar levels. Certain chemicals in our brains – referred to as opiates – have been linked to feeling happy and are often dubbed 'feel-good' chemicals. The best known are the endorphins – the natural painkillers that give rise to the 'runner's high' experienced by athletes.

In his book *Breaking the Food Seduction*, Dr Neal Barnard says that sugar causes the release of natural opiates, 'cousins of morphine and heroin' in terms of chemical structure. The result is, he says, 'whatever physical or psychological troubles might have been bothering you are toned down a bit'. In other words, the opiate-releasing effect of sugar can make you feel like nothing else matters.

To complicate the situation, sugar and other foods rich in refined carbohydrates are also responsible for boosting levels of serotonin, another brain chemical which helps regulate mood and sleep. The release of serotonin that comes from eating sugar brings with it feelings of contentment and relaxation.

The trouble is that if you're hooked on sugar, you need it to feel good. Low beta-endorphin levels can leave you with cravings and low self-esteem, while low serotonin levels can result in depression. Other experts say if you don't have a sugar 'fix', you suffer withdrawal symptoms and can start to feel irritable. Most sugar addicts will respond to this by feeding the addiction, simply so they can feel 'normal' again. But the relief they get is only temporary, and this just locks them further into sugar addiction.

Professor Marie Reid counters that feeling better after eating sugary foods is more likely down to 'reinforcement' – *believing* that the food makes you feel better – rather than its impact on serotonin.

Nicki's Emotional Addiction
'For me, sugar is associated with wonderful thoughts and happy memories. When I used to think of it, I felt contented. And looking back on my idyllic childhood, I understand why. Food – especially sweet food – was given to me with unconditional love and care. Each week, my grandmother would bring me freshly made fudge or toffee and it'd be handed to me with a big kiss and a hug.

'My other grandmother also baked the most wonderful cakes – apple cake, marble cake, cheesecake – and the family would all sit down to enjoy them together. I remember going to the funfair with my parents and always having pink candyfloss and pink and white nougat. But perhaps most significant was what I did every Saturday morning, without fail, with my best mate, Tania. We'd pool our pocket money which we'd be given as a reward if we'd behaved and done all our homework that week. We'd then cycle down to the corner shop to spend the lot on pick 'n' mix. We'd put it all on the bedroom floor and spend the entire morning playing with our dolls and working our way through our stash of sweets. We were both in heaven!

'Also, every day after school, we took it in turns to go back to each other's homes for tea and there would always be buttered toast with jam, French fancies, jam tarts and Wagon Wheels on the menu. Sugary foods were what I ate on happy family gatherings, fun times with my best friend and as a reward for being a good girl. How could sugar be a bad thing when it had so many good associations?

'As a result, sugar became a sure-fire way of making me feel happy. Even if things were going wrong in my life, I knew I could always get a high – however temporary – from eating sugar. It took me back to those "happy places" of my childhood. But as all sugar addicts know, this love of sugar – wherever it stems from – comes at a price.

'In many ways, my overwhelming desire to eat sweet foods felt physical – I'd experience the sugar highs and lows throughout the day as a matter of course, and would reach for sugary foods to keep me feeling balanced. But there's no doubt in my mind that my sugar addiction had extremely strong emotional roots, too, stemming from positive childhood messages about sweet foods. I also know I have an addictive personality, which doesn't help in my fight to do things in moderation – including cutting back on sugar. In my experience, beating sugar addiction needs a two-pronged approach. You need to work at the physical side, through nutrition and exercise, but understand when, where and why the emotional side starts kicking in, too.'

GETTING OVER YOUR ADDICTION

As well as offering psychological support, experts who help people overcome eating disorders encourage their patients to return to eating regular meals based on complex carbohydrates and protein. These foods satisfy hunger and provide slow-release energy. Patients get into the habit of eating properly to satisfy their emotional needs but also to help stabilize blood-sugar levels and prevent the need to binge on sweet or refined foods.

Nicki's diet works on these principles – regular eating of the right foods to keep you from bingeing on sugary foods, plus keeping a food diary to get you more in tune with your eating habits.

Keeping a Diary

When you get to the 21-day plan (Chapter 13), you'll see that the first day's task is to start keeping a food diary.

So why are we asking you to keep a food diary? Most of us eat food without thinking about how it makes us feel – it's just like fuel to fill our faces and stomachs. But it is important to know what you're eating and how it makes you feel. For starters, if you're not clued up about food, you can end up eating more than you should, the wrong types of food or going a day eating hardly anything. Actions like these can lead to weight gain and feelings of illness and/or unhappiness. Writing it down in a diary helps you to take a good, hard look at your eating habits. Also, if you don't write it down, it's easy to forget that mini chocolate bar you ate, or the half portion of chips you finished off your kids' plates!

There is an example of Nicki's food diary on page 53. Nicki found that filling in the diary helped her understand the times of the day when her cravings were at their worst (such as on waking and the 'post-lunch' dip), and aware of foods that made her happy or short-tempered, satisfied or bloated. Working from left to right, these are the columns to be filled in:

- **Time of day** – put in WHEN you ate.
- **Food/Drink** – fill in WHAT you ate. Put exactly what you ate (e.g. one large baked potato with tuna and sweetcorn, NOT just 'jacket potato').

- **Physical symptoms** – write in how you felt PHYSICALLY (e.g. rushed, sick, hungry, full).
- **How you're feeling** – put in how you felt EMOTIONALLY (happy, grumpy, tearful, normal). For ideas of how you might feel (rather than just filling in 'fine') see our list below.
- **Other factors**. Here you might want to put in such things as 'Have PMS' or 'Had argument with colleague' or even 'First day of holiday' – anything that may be relevant to the choices you're making and how you're feeling. Also record your exercise here. Don't forget it's not just the gym that counts. 'Walking the dog' goes in here, too!

How You're Feeling: Some Suggestions

PHYSICAL SYMPTOMS: POSITIVE
Full of energy/energized
Clear skin
Bright eyes
Satisfied (just enough food!)
Relaxed
Pain-free

EMOTIONAL SYMPTOMS: POSITIVE
Happy
Clever
Beautiful

Calm
Contented
Positive
Grounded
Confident
Proud
Strong
Pleased
Bubbly
Popular

PHYSICAL SYMPTOMS: NEGATIVE
Bloated
Constipated
Indigestion
Headache
In pain
Tired
Drowsy
Poor concentration
Spotty
Bad skin
Trouble sleeping
Gained weight
PMS
Toxic

EMOTIONAL SYMPTOMS: NEGATIVE
Negative
Sad
Restless
Knackered!
Depressed
Angry
Grumpy
Fed up
Blue
Bored
Impatient
Ratty
Jumpy
High
Anxious

What to Look Out for in Your Food Diary
At the end of each day, take a look at your food diary to see exactly what you've eaten. Turn to Chapter 8 and see which list you've picked most of your foods from: 'Foods you can eat', 'Occasional treats' or 'Foods to avoid'. It might help you to photocopy these pages for quick reference or mark them with a sticky note so you can quickly flip to them. Don't be down if you've picked most from the 'Foods to avoid' list – that's what happened to Nicki, too! The aim of this book is to show you how you can make choices from the 'Foods you can

eat' list (plus occasional treats) without feeling like you've been hard done by.

After a few days, you may start to see patterns. Look for the following:

- Are you eating regularly?
- Are you eating at least five portions of fruit and veg a day?
- Are you having sweet snacks?
- Do you have sugary drinks (e.g. canned fizzy drinks)?
- Are you doing any exercise?
- How many hours do you spend watching TV each day?

It could well be that you start to see things in your eating habits that you never noticed before. With this information, you'll start to build up a picture of how you eat, why you eat, when you eat and what bad habits you may have got into. Don't worry – we're going to help you put these right.

Nicki's Diary: How She Used to Eat

Here's an example of Nicki's food diary to help you see how it might look. You'll notice that in some boxes she puts just one word and in others she puts more. This is down to personal choice – do what you think will help you most.

Why We Crave Sugar

TIME OF DAY	FOOD/ DRINK	PHYSICAL SYMPTOMS	HOW YOU'RE FEELING	OTHER FACTORS
8am	White baguette with cheese Plain croissant Cup of tea with sweetener	Full	A bit Tense	Big work day ahead - stress!
10.30 am	Haven't Eaten	Dizzy, Weak	Edgy!	
11.15 am	Pick 'n' mix (two handfulls)	Full of Energy	Happy	
11.30 pm		Tired	Edgy, A bit sad	
1 pm	Half a cheese Sandwich and cup of tea	Hungry, then full and bloated	A bit low (don't like being bloated)	Didn't have time for proper lunch
2 pm	more Pick 'n' mix	Hunger pangs beginning	Happy	
2.15 pm		Lacking Energy, headachey	Low	Doing a Workout
3.30 pm	Cup of tea Packet of crisps Kit-Kat	Hungry then full (but hungry again half an hour later	Grumpy!	
7.30 pm	Salmon Steak, new potatoes, courgettes Yoghurt with fruit	Light-headed then properly full for the first time today	Contented	First proper meal for almost 12 hours
9.30 pm	Bowl of porridge with sultanas	Peckish but not with a rumbling tummy!	Still feeling happy	

SUGAR ADDICTS' DIET

The times listed reflect Nicki's routine at the time. Yours might be different – for example, you might have breakfast at 6am or perhaps you don't have it at all! If you skip a meal, you should still write it in because it will provide you with important information about how this makes you feel physically and emotionally. Don't forget to put the date at the top of each diary day. And if you're feeling lazy and are tempted to let the whole diary thing slip, remember this: weight management experts say that people who don't keep a regular food diary don't tend to lose weight. One study found that heavier women were also more likely to under-report their daily food intake than those who were lean, so if you're reading this book to lose weight, the diary will help you stop kidding yourself about how much you're eating!

From this we can see:

- When Nicki didn't eat, she felt dizzy, weak and edgy.
- When she ate something really sugary, like pick 'n' mix, she felt happy and full of energy. But just 15 minutes later, she felt tired, edgy and a bit sad (as soon as the sugar 'high' has worn off).
- When she didn't eat a proper lunch, she needed another sugar lift within an hour, suggesting that her blood sugar levels were low. The result? She went for the sweets again.
- When she grabbed a lunch, it didn't satisfy her for long and she ended up having crisps and chocolate to stave off her hunger mid-afternoon.

Why We Crave Sugar

- It was only following a proper meal at 7.30pm that she felt 'contented' – and continued to feel happy a couple of hours later.
- We could also see that she wasn't eating enough fruit and veg.
- On a more positive note, she was getting some exercise, wasn't watching hours of telly and wasn't having fizzy drinks.

This was Nicki's eating regime before she started the Sugar Addicts' Diet. By looking at this diary, Nicki was able to see exactly how the foods she ate affected her physically and emotionally. By filling in your own diary, you can do the same. You don't have to do it forever, but try to keep it going for at least the 21 days of the plan.

Nicki says, 'I've eaten like this for years, and until I wrote it down, I had no idea of how food could affect how I felt. Now I can see how certain foods affect me – for good and for bad – I can decide what to go for and what to avoid. I hate feeling 'low', 'edgy', 'grumpy' and all those other negative words. I only ever want to put positive words in the diary!'

4
Why Do I Need to Break My Addiction?

So you're addicted to sugar – what's the problem with that? Well, for starters, if you're reading a book with the word 'diet' in the title, it's likely you're carrying an extra pound or two. In other words, you need to lose some weight. For many people, this is their first reason for wanting to overcome their love of sugar. There is a range of other medical conditions that are aggravated or even caused by eating too much sugar. The sugar industry disputes this and, to be fair, we'll tell you what they say so you can make your own mind up. We think the facts speak for themselves but it's up to you to decide whether you think the pursuit of giving up sugar is a worthwhile one.

OVERWEIGHT AND OBESITY
- Nearly two-thirds of men and over half of all women in the UK are now overweight
- One in five of us is obese – at least 2–3 stones overweight

SUGAR ADDICTS' DIET

- Two-thirds of adults over 45 are overweight or obese
- Almost 1 in 10 6-year-olds and almost 1 in 6 15-year-olds is obese
- Obesity is linked to around 30,000 deaths a year through heart disease, strokes and diabetes

As you can see, obesity is a huge problem in the UK, and it's on the increase all over the world. The level of obesity has gone up three times in the past 20 years, and it's still rising. At this rate, one in four adults will be obese by 2010 and one in three by 2020. Just imagine it – as you sit with two of your friends or family members, one of you will be not just overweight but obese.

But excess weight doesn't just mean not being able to fit into the clothes you want – it can seriously affect your health, too. Among other things, it puts us at greater risk of diabetes, osteoarthritis, high blood pressure, coronary heart disease, stroke and some cancers. In fact, recent reports suggest that obesity may soon overtake cigarette smoking as a serious health risk. The International Obesity Task Force estimates that 1.7 billion people across the world may be at risk of weight-related health problems.

The standard measurement for weight is the body mass index (BMI), which is weight in kilograms divided by height in metres squared:

$$BMI = \frac{weight\ (kg)}{height\ (m) \times height\ (m)}$$

Why Do I Need to Break My Addiction?

For example, if you weigh 10 stone and you are 5 feet 6 inches tall, you would work out your BMI by finding your weight in kilos (63kg) and your height in metres (1.68m):

$$BMI = \frac{63kg}{(1.68m \times 1.68m)\ 2.8m} = 22.5$$

Overweight is a BMI of 25–30 while obese is 30–40. So, for example, someone 5 feet 6 inches tall (1.68m) becomes obese at 13 stone 4 pounds (84kg) and morbidly obese at 17 stones 7 pounds (110kg). Obesity becomes 'morbid' when it significantly increases the risk of one or more obesity-related health conditions or serious diseases.

A simpler way of measuring your health, however, is by your waistline. The World Health Organization recommends a limit for waist circumference of 102cm and 88cm in men and women respectively. Want to know how to measure yourself and what this means? Visit the National Obesity Forum's Waist Watch Action Campaign website at www.nationalobesityforum.org.uk and visit the Public Info area.

The Role of Sugar

You'd be hard-pressed to find a doctor who'll say a diet high in sugar is a good thing and doesn't increase your risk of putting on weight. The problem is that high sugar consumption coupled with increasingly low activity levels (as we now have in the UK) equals weight gain. Recent research published in the British Medical Journal found that when children avoided cans of pop, obesity levels fell, but it rose among those who kept on drinking them. Excess sugar consumption can increase insulin levels, leading to overweight and obesity plus an increased risk of Type 2 diabetes and other conditions we'll tell you about in this chapter.

DIABETES
- Diabetes affects 1.4 million people in England
- Diabetes UK says there may be as many as another million people who have diabetes but don't realize it – the 'missing million'
- The number of people being diagnosed with diabetes increases each year
- It's estimated that five per cent of all NHS expenditure is on diabetes

Type 2 diabetes is where the body fails to produce enough insulin or doesn't know how to use the insulin it has made. It used to be called 'late' or 'adult onset' diabetes because the average age of diagnosis is around 52. But **rising levels of obesity has led to Type 2 diabetes being seen increasingly in younger people – even children.**

Why Do I Need to Break My Addiction?

Diabetes UK says the fact that as a nation we are increasingly overweight and less active is key to the rise in diabetes. Central body fat – being 'apple shaped' – is strongly linked to insulin resistance, where the body produces insulin but isn't able to use it properly. Studies show that diabetes increases the risk of ill health from conditions such as heart disease, stroke and kidney failure and shortens lifespan. One study says Type 2 diabetes doubles or trebles the risk of dying prematurely.

The Role of Sugar
Although laboratory studies have failed to show a direct link between diabetes and normal sugar consumption, diabetes *is* linked to obesity which is, in turn, linked to sugar. And as our nation gets fatter, so our levels of Type 2 diabetes increase. Also, very high levels of sugar consumption (more than 200g per day) are considered a possible risk factor for developing diabetes.

SYNDROME X
Research at Leeds Metropolitan University in 2002 revealed that one in five British people may suffer from a condition called Syndrome X (also known as 'sugar overload disorder'). With this condition, sufferers have constantly high blood-sugar levels because of a sugary diet. As a result, they have raised levels of fats (triglycerides) but low levels of 'good' HDL cholesterol in the blood, which increases the risk of heart disease.

Importantly, they also have **insulin resistance** where the sugar-regulating hormone insulin becomes less capable of removing glucose from the blood. Instead it is stored as fat around the waist and upper body.

The result? If untreated, there's an increased risk of developing Type 2 (adult-onset) diabetes, obesity and high blood pressure. Professor Gerald Reaven of Stanford University, California, first coined the term Syndrome X in 1988. He called it the 'silent killer' because its early stages often go unnoticed and many people don't even know they have it.

The Role of Sugar

Dr Victor Zammit of the Hannah Research Institute in Ayr, Scotland, has discovered that Syndrome X may be linked to high-calorie sugary snacks and drinks. If eaten often enough, these high-sugar foods can lead to constantly raised insulin levels without giving the body a break in between. Eventually, this overwork may hinder the ability of the pancreas to produce sufficient insulin, leading to problems such as Type 2 diabetes.

In his book *Fat Land*, Greg Critser uses the 'doorbell analogy' to describe this breakdown – '... it would be as if one constantly rang one's neighbour's doorbell and then ran away; eventually the neighbour would stop coming to the door'. In other words, after overproducing insulin to cope with constantly high sugar levels, eventually the pancreas will stop bothering. A diet high in hidden sugar and refined carbohydrates can also lead to Syndrome X and further complications. Excess fat can make insulin resistance worse and cause insulin levels to rise.

CANCER

- One in three people will be diagnosed with cancer during their lifetime
- It is estimated that one-third of all cancers are caused by diet
- Bowel cancer is the second most common cancer in women, with 16,800 new cases being diagnosed each year
- Researchers predict that the rise in obesity and overweight will cause cancer rates to soar by 50 per cent worldwide by 2020

A report by the World Health Organization's International Agency for Research on Cancer estimates that being overweight and inactive accounts for one-fifth to one-third of all breast, colon, endometrial, kidney and oesophageal cancers. Eating habits are also thought to influence risk of bowel, mouth, stomach and pancreatic cancer, and may also be a risk factor for prostate, lung, cervical and bladder cancer. **The advice of Cancer Research UK is to eat a healthy and balanced diet including plenty of fruit and veg, high-fibre foods, starchy foods like potatoes and lower levels of fat and red or processed meat.**

The Role of Sugar

Obesity is directly linked to cancer, and a diet high in sugar increases the likelihood of weight gain (possibly to the point of obesity). Researchers in America say that excess fat can act as a continuous 'hormone pump', leading to changes in the body that create favourable conditions for cancer to begin.

Other studies, however, make a more direct link between sugar consumption and cancer. One US study of more than 38,000 women, reported in the *Journal of the National Cancer Institute*, suggested a link between a diet high in sugar and colorectal cancer. The risk was almost three times higher in women with the highest dietary glycaemic load (in other words, those who ate more foods with a higher glycaemic index, see page 40).

Another study, this time at the University of Minnesota, indicated that women with a higher dietary glycaemic load may be at greater risk of developing cancer of the womb. American author Dr Patrick Quillin says that eating foods that keep blood-sugar levels balanced is vital for cancer patients and advisable for those who don't have cancer. In his book *Beating Cancer with Nutrition* he says, 'Elevating blood glucose in a cancer patient is like throwing gasoline on a smouldering fire.'

HEART AND CIRCULATION DISEASES
- Heart and circulatory diseases are the UK's biggest killer
- Coronary heart disease accounts for one in six deaths in women and one in four in men
- Heart disease is an increasing problem in the UK, not least because of rising levels of obesity and overweight, which put a strain on the heart and circulatory system. As we've already seen, being overweight also increases the risk of developing Type 2 diabetes (page 60), which brings with it an increased risk of heart problems.

The Role of Sugar
A diet persistently high in sugar means blood-sugar levels that are constantly raised above normal levels. High sugar levels raise the levels of serum triglycerides (fat in the blood) and harmful very low density lipoproteins (VLDL) – both risk factors for atherosclerosis, or furring up of the arteries. High blood-sugar levels trigger the release of more insulin into the bloodstream, and insulin increases the risk of arteriosclerotic plaques on the walls of blood vessels.

POLYCYSTIC OVARIAN SYNDROME (PCOS)
Polycystic ovaries are when a woman develops many small follicles (cysts) in her ovaries which can hinder monthly ovulation. About 1 in 10 UK women have

polycystic ovaries to some degree, and PCOS is found in around 70 per cent of women who have ovulation difficulties leading to infertility. Many women with PCOS are found to be insulin resistant so it's thought this plays a major part in the condition. The body produces more insulin than normal in an attempt to reduce blood-sugar levels but this extra insulin (along with the testosterone it also stimulates) stops follicles developing and prevents ovulation.

The Role of Sugar
A high-sugar diet can aggravate PCOS by increasing blood insulin levels and keeping them at a constantly raised level. PCOS can be worsened by overweight and obesity because excess fat can cause insulin levels to rise and make the resistance worse. However, PCOS can also contribute to overweight and obesity – a bit of a 'catch-22' situation. Good general advice to sufferers is to cut back on added sugars and refined carbohydrates.

CANDIDA
Candida occurs when yeast that is naturally present in our bodies changes into its fungal form, travels through the gut walls and leads to toxins entering the bloodstream. This can produce a wide range of symptoms, from food cravings and allergies to depression. Blood-sugar imbalances – such as diabetes and low blood-sugar levels

Why Do I Need to Break My Addiction?

(hypoglycaemia) – can prompt Candida to multiply and cause problems.

The Role of Sugar
An overly sugary diet feeds the yeast at the root of the problem. Candida thrives on sugar so if you are prone to yeast infections, it's important to reduce the amount of sugary foods and refined carbohydrates in your diet. Craving sweet foods is often a sign of Candida. If you think you might have Candida, you should seek advice from a doctor or nutritionist who may advise tests and an elimination diet to confirm the cause and tackle it.

DIGESTIVE PROBLEMS
- One in ten British people suffers from a digestive disorder
- Digestive disorders account for around one in sixteen deaths

Whether we're talking about gallbladder problems, bloating or flatulence, digestive disorders can be painful, miserable or simply inconvenient. What we eat directly influences the health of our digestive systems.

The Role of Sugar
Sugar and other refined carbohydrates can cause real problems for the digestive system. The refined carbs cling to the gut wall where they feed unwanted gut

bacteria, helping it to thrive instead of passing out of the body. These bacteria lead to inflammation in the gut and an immune response. If the immune response goes on for too long – as it can do if the diet is constantly high in sugar and refined carbs – the body may start to produce too much insulin. In other words, you could become 'insulin resistant' and end up with health problems such as Type 2 diabetes, heart disease, obesity, PCOS, high blood pressure or even arthritis.

TOOTH DECAY
- Eating a diet high in sugar increases the risk of tooth decay
- 53 per cent of children have decay in their permanent or primary teeth
- Drinking fizzy drinks increases the chance of tooth decay in 12-year-olds by 59 per cent. Four or more glasses daily increases the risk by 252 per cent

The role of sugar in causing tooth decay has been known for hundreds of years. Queen Elizabeth I had terrible tooth decay after sucking on bars of the 'white gold' (as sugar used to be known). In its 2003 World Oral Health Report, the World Health Organization announced that dental problems such as tooth decay and gum disease are on the rise, and one of the major reasons is our ever increasing love of sugar. One survey found that thousands of children under the age of five are having large numbers of milk teeth removed in hospital because they are so badly decayed.

The Role of Sugar

Tooth decay happens when bacteria in your mouth use sugar from food to make acids. Over time, these acids can create holes or cavities in the tooth – decayed areas that require treatment such as fillings or even removal of teeth. When it comes to tooth decay in children, Professor Aubrey Sheiham, Professor of Dental Public Health at University College London, says, 'Some people think, "They're only baby teeth – what does it matter." But that doesn't take into account the impact of pain and suffering that goes with tooth decay.'

Tooth decay can lead to problems with eating and chewing, dental abscesses and missing or damaged teeth – something that can cause distress well into adulthood. There are socio-economic implications, too – decay can mean children miss school and parents have to take time off work to look after them. Perhaps most significantly, studies now show that decayed teeth can retard growth in children. Professor Sheiham says, 'Pain, inflammation or abscesses mean children can end up eating softer foods which might not be so nutritious, and this can have an impact on their growth.'

DEPRESSION
- Depression is one of the most common medical conditions in Britain today
- One in five British people will be affected by depression at some stage in their life
- More than 2.9 million people in the UK are diagnosed with depression
- The World Health Organization predicts depression will be second only to heart disease as the biggest global health burden by 2020
- As many as three in four cases of depression are neither recognized nor treated

The Role of Sugar
If you're feeling blue, reaching for sugar may be your first thought. But you could be doing yourself a great disservice. While sugar causes the release of 'feel-good' endorphins, the payback is when we come down from that 'high', often into feelings of depression. Professor Larry Christenden at the University of South Alabama found that drastically cutting down on sugar lifted depression in 25 per cent of patients. He says that while carbohydrates can produce mood-lifting serotonin in the brain, it could be that some people have a negative reaction to pure sugar, making them depressed.

ACNE

Acne is generally associated with increased levels of the male sex hormone testosterone, which is why it's common in puberty (there's an increase in testosterone in both sexes at this time). It is also found in women with polycystic ovaries (see page 65) where an imbalance in the female sex hormones leads to an increased production of testosterone by the ovaries.

The Role of Sugar

Experts say that poor glucose metabolism is one of the causes of acne. Professor Loren Cordain of Colorado State University says the Western diet of refined sugars and starches may be to blame for high rates of acne. These foods produce high levels of insulin, which in turn produces testosterone and the overproduction of pore-blocking sebum.

AND THERE'S MORE!

The list of sugar-related ailments doesn't end there. High levels of sugar in the diet have also been linked to:

- **Ageing**. Sugar interacts with collagen in a reaction called glycosylation. This reaction makes the skin inflexible and robs it of its natural plumpness. The result? An increased risk of ageing and wrinkly skin.
- **Pain and inflammation**. These can be caused by disturbed blood-sugar control.

- **Immunity problems.** Sugars increase our body's production of the 'fight or flight' hormone, adrenaline, by four times. This increases the production of cortisone which reduces immunity, leaving the path nice and clear for colds, chest infections and sore throats. It also reduces the production of antibodies which 'fight' invaders, and interferes with vitamin C transport (an important nutrient for immune function).
- **Vaginal yeast infections.** As well as feeding Candida (see above), sugar also feeds the yeast that can lead to vaginal thrush. More than half of all women have at least one bout of thrush in their life.
- **PMS symptoms.** According to a report in the Journal of Reproductive Medicine, women who said they had PMS symptoms consumed three times the amount of sugar as those who didn't have symptoms. PMS is associated with blood-sugar imbalances.

WHAT THE SUGAR INDUSTRY TELLS YOU

The sugar industry is worth billions of pounds internationally every year. Not surprising, really, when you see how sugar seems to be in so many types of food, both sweet and savoury. As a result, the sugar lobby (those in charge of promoting and 'selling' it) goes to great lengths to tell you it's really not as bad as people think it is. In fact, the US sugar industry threatened to withdraw its £260m funding of the World Health

Why Do I Need to Break My Addiction?

Organization when the WHO issued healthy-eating guidelines. Specifically, the sugar industry objected to the recommendation that no more than 10 per cent of our daily energy should come from extrinsic (added) sugars.

Here are some of the things the sugar industry says about sugar and health:

'Sugar is natural'

Just because something is natural, it doesn't mean to say you can eat it in abundance. Lots of fats are natural, too, but we're not telling you to eat lots of those, either.

'Sugar may help people stick to slimming diets'

Does sugar make you fat? The sugar industry points to studies which suggest that slim people tend to eat more sugar while overweight people eat less sugar but more fat. In other words, they say fat is the main culprit. A 1998 World Health Organization report also suggests that a balanced diet that includes sugar together with physical activity helps prevent obesity. But before you rest on your laurels and say, 'Well, that must mean I can carry on eating sugar', look at these facts in context. Sure, a slim person might be able to eat more sugar and not put on weight but their bodies can cope with this because they generally have other healthy habits, such as exercising regularly, to counteract it. A little sugar is, indeed, fine as part of a balanced, active life (our brains need carbohydrates to break down into glucose to function) but the fact is that the majority of us don't live this way. We eat too much and exercise too little.

'Sugar makes food taste good'

Of course it does, but it's possible to enjoy food without piling heaps of sugar onto it. If you like that sweet taste, there's no reason why you shouldn't have it, but get it from a source that's better for your health – fruit. Fruit has intrinsic sugar which your body copes with much better than extrinsic 'added' sugars. Sugary foods are often made to taste better by the addition of fat, so if you're tasting sugar in a processed food such as biscuits or chocolate, chances are you're also eating more fat than you really should be. So yes, it tastes good – but at a price!

'Active people need sugar'

Yes, they do. If we're active, eating carbs will provide our muscles with energy. Carbs are also the brain's first choice as an energy source. If you are physically active, it's therefore important to have carbohydrates. But before you say, 'I go to the gym three times a week' or 'I have a physically demanding job', we're still not talking about you. When we say 'active' we mean people like professional athletes who are using the sugar as part of a strict training regime.

Dr Sarah Schenker, nutrition scientist at the British Nutrition Foundation, says, 'Athletes have sugar as part

Why Do I Need to Break My Addiction?

of their diets but they eat a very strict diet where exact amounts and even the time when they eat are taken into account. The rest of us who live in the real world simply don't eat like that – and we don't need the sugar they do.'

The majority of us get all the sugar we need from a well-balanced diet containing good-quality complex carbohydrates. As you'll see in the next chapter, some carbohydrates give a more steady release of glucose than others. For most of us, there's simply no need to pile on the white stuff, too!

5

Young Sugar Addicts

FAT KIDS: THE BARE FACTS
- Almost one in ten six-year-olds and almost one in six 15-year-olds is obese
- There was a 140 per cent increase in obesity in primary-school children between 1984 and 1994
- In 1974, 7 per cent of children aged 7–11 were overweight – by 2002 that figure was 27 per cent
- Children's waistlines have expanded by two clothing sizes (4cm) in two decades
- Most children have higher intakes of saturated fats, sugar and salt than the maximum recommended for adults
- If current trends continue, at least a fifth of boys and a third of girls will be obese by 2020
- More than half of all 4–18-year-olds have some decay in either their milk teeth or permanent teeth

Imagine your six-year-old in a class of 30 children. According to these statistics, three of their classmates will be obese. British children are fatter than ever before.

The emotional impact of being an overweight child is well-documented – chubby children are more likely to be bullied. Children's anti-bullying charity Kidscape says victims of chronic bullying are seven times more likely to suffer depression in later life and attempt suicide.

The physical impacts are equally worrying. The Food Standards Agency has warned that poor nutrition and lack of exercise means young people today are on average likely to live shorter lives than their parents – the first such reduction in more than a century. Dr Colin Waine of the National Obesity Forum says fat kids have an up to 20 per cent greater risk of developing cancer as adults.

On a very simple level, children now eat more and are less active than kids a generation before them. But when it comes to doing something about it, it isn't as easy as saying 'eat less and exercise more'. It's not just us adults who are being bombarded with messages about food from advertisers – it's happening to kids, too. And if we are to reverse this trend of childhood obesity, we need to look at the 'whole package', not just exercise and healthy eating.

There's a growing awareness of how much food manufacturers, advertisers and even schools are adding to the burden of bad diets and obesity in children. The Children's Food Bill, put before Parliament in May 2004, is calling for legislation to protect children from junk-food marketing, as well as calling for improvements in food education in schools, and better-quality school food. In 2004, the Consumers' Association published its Health Warning to Government in which it made 12 demands to help address the obesity crisis. One of these demands is that the big four high-street supermarkets develop a labelling scheme to help consumers easily identify foods high in sugar, fat and salt. Some food manufacturers, who have long insisted they're not to blame, are talking about introducing subtle changes to their products – in July 2003, Kraft (which produces Dairylea and Toblerone) pledged to scale down its portions and reduce sugar and salt levels. But experts argue there's still a long way to go and we've only just begun to take the issue of childhood obesity seriously.

In the next chapter, we'll be giving advice on how to help kids resist influences that encourage them to eat badly and to guide them towards healthier eating choices. But before that, we'll take a look at where these messages come from and what they mean for our kids. We're also going to draw on Nicki's experiences of helping kids to develop better habits in Inch Loss Juniors so you can give your own children a fighting chance in the battle against sugar addiction and obesity.

WHY ARE KIDS EATING UNHEALTHY FOODS?
The Growth of Special 'Children's Foods'

There are certain foods we probably all associate with being a child, such as candy floss, sweets such as jelly babies and ice creams. Without the need for fancy, persuasive adverts, they've been viewed as 'children's foods' for decades. But in the past 20 years, there has been an increasing trend towards manufacturing and marketing foods for children. Children's foods now include snacks and savoury foods such as Dairylea Lunchables, Heinz Thomas the Tank Engine and Friends pasta and cereals such as Scooby Doo chocolate-flavoured cereal and Kellogg's Disney Hunny Bs with Piglet biscuits. This is just the tip of the iceberg – supermarkets are full of foods made into the shapes of fish, faces or even dinosaurs to appeal to children. This is all very well, but often these foods are highly processed, containing high levels of sugar and salt that help to bump up daily intakes beyond recommended amounts.

These less desirable foods also tend to replace healthier options. Nutritionist Dr Helen Crawley analysed two daily menus of food that a child might eat, based on those that are specifically marketed at them. She concluded that 'to follow either diet on a regular basis would be damaging to a child's health', and that it could increase the risk of tooth decay, overweight, diabetes, cancers and heart disease in later life.

Advertising

- Seventy per cent of parents say there should be no advertising of junk foods during kids' television viewing times
- Food and drinks firms place 30–56 per cent of their commercials during programmes aimed at youngsters

Children now spend more time in front of the telly than ever before, an average of six hours a day. But they're not just viewing programmes – they're watching adverts, too. One study found that adverts during children's programmes are mainly for foods of little nutritional value. A report by Sustain, a pressure group campaigning to protect children from unhealthy advertising, found that during children's viewing times, up to 99 per cent of food and drink products advertised contained high levels of fat, sugar and salt, and the largest category of advertised food was sweets, cakes and biscuits. In fact, if a child was to eat all the fatty and sugary foods advertised during this time, they'd be consuming 11 times the recommended intake for kids. Not only that, but while they're watching television on Saturday mornings, kids are subjected to twice as many adverts per hour for unhealthy foods as adults are after the 9pm watershed.

Looked at like this, it's no wonder our children are so keen on fatty, sugary foods. Experts say there is 'selective targeting of children by promoters of unhealthy foods'. In other words, **our kids are being singled out by advertisers who know they're an easy target**. The problem is food advertising on television encourages both obese and non-obese children to eat more and to eat more unhealthily, according to a recent study from Liverpool University.

Entertainment

When you watch a film, you may or may not be aware of how much 'product placement' there is. Whether it's flash cars, expensive watches or even branded cigarettes, manufacturers will have paid huge sums of money to film companies to showcase their products. The same happens with food and drinks. And when children see this, it influences how they act and feel.

In one study, children aged 6–12 were shown a clip of the movie *Home Alone*. One half of the group was shown a scene in which Pepsi Cola was mentioned, while the other half saw a similar scene with food and milk but no branded products. When the children were later asked to help themselves to a soft drink – either Coke or Pepsi – those exposed to the 'branded' clip were significantly more likely to choose Pepsi. Researchers also found that when the children were interviewed later, many of those who chose Pepsi couldn't recall having seen the brand on screen.

Fast food and soft drinks have also been found frequently in children's films. *Teenage Mutant Ninja*

Turtles features Domino's Pizzas, while Burger King, McDonald's, Pizza Hut, Coca-Cola and Pepsi have appeared in films such as *Gremlins, Mac and Me, Back to the Future II* and *Big*.

Celebrity Endorsement

- 82 per cent of parents think celebrity endorsements have a considerable influence on children's food choices

We Brits are obsessed with celebrities. We want to know all about them, including where they go on holiday, what they buy and what they like to eat. As a result, if we see one of them using a product or eating or drinking a particular food, we want it, too. Perhaps we think it will help us to achieve their enviable lifestyle.

It's not just adults that fall for this – kids do, too, which is why advertisers are so keen to get celebrities to promote their products. Footballer Gary Lineker and pop star Victoria Beckham have both advertised Walker's crisps; supermodels Caprice, Cindy Crawford and Linda Evangelista have all advertised Pizza Hut; and Britney Spears and Robbie Williams have been involved in ad campaigns for Pepsi.

The respected medical journal, *The Lancet*, said celebrity endorsement of junk food should be banned because it contributes to high rates of obesity, especially in children. The impact of these celebrities urging us to buy is so powerful that it has been suggested there should be laws to prevent firms from using celebrities to endorse products high in fat, sugar and salt. It was also recently proposed that celebrities be used to endorse healthy foods instead of junk. Until this happens, children's poor food choices continue to be influenced by their sporting, musical or movie heroes in ad campaigns.

Shopping

Every parent knows how shopping for food with a child can be exhausting ... because of 'pester power'. Kids are increasingly influenced by the likes of advertising and celebrity endorsement, and when they see food products they recognize because of these, they have to have them.

The fact your children want these foods is no accident. It's part of a very clever strategy. A survey carried out by the Consumers' Association criticized food and drink manufacturers for the tactics used to sell their products to children. Offering free gifts and targeting schools to promote goods is commonplace. In fact, UK companies are spending an estimated £300 million a year on targeting schools with endorsement deals, such as sports equipment in exchange for food wrappers. Nicki says: 'As a trainer, I'm all for things that increase people's opportunity to get active, but I think this is a case of "robbing Peter to pay Paul". Yes, the kids might benefit from sports equipment, but they have to stuff their faces with poor quality food to get hold of it in the first place!'

Young Sugar Addicts

In a recent report, food watchdog the Food Commission said that junk food advertisers know that children easily fall for marketing messages and they target children as young as two with offers such as free toys. In the Consumers' Association survey, **more than three-quarters of parents felt that free gifts such as toys that come with McDonald's Happy Meals, or collectable items in breakfast cereals, influence their children to want particular foods**. And as most parents will tell you, this 'pester power' is hard to ignore! Other marketing techniques used by food and drink manufacturers to get you to buy are gimmicky packaging, the use of cartoon characters (such as Tony the Tiger and the Honey Monster who are used to sell breakfast cereals) and interactive websites to develop brand loyalty. The trouble is that when the reason for the sale is something like packaging or branding, kids aren't bothered whether the food itself is healthy or not.

Peer Pressure

Most of us can remember school friends who always seemed to have nicer food in their lunch box than we did. Nicki says, 'I hear stories all the time of "lunch box envy". Kids feel that what they bring in for lunch helps make them more popular, if it's a new or exciting food product. The other side of the coin is that they're embarrassed to be seen eating healthy food and feel it could even make friends think less of them.' Sussex paediatric dietician Heidi Guy agrees that kids are under pressure to be seen eating the 'right' foods by friends. She says children are even bullied in the playground over brands of food in their lunch box. But it's food in bright, colourful packaging that's so often the highest in fat and sugar, not to mention additives such as colourings, flavourings and preservatives.

Family Influence
Let's get something straight – we're not 'parent bashing' here. As a mum of two children herself, Nicki knows only too well how hard it can be to make the right choices for kids. She says, 'As a parent, I know only too well how confusing it can all be. You're treading a fine line between making food an issue by giving them things they don't want and buying them rubbish food they want because they've seen it on TV or they've eaten it at a friend's house. There's also so much conflicting information out there. One minute we're told something is good for our kids, the next a study comes out saying it could be harmful. No wonder parents are often confused beyond belief.'

Many parents admit that they're worried about the way their kids' eating is being influenced by advertising – in a government poll, 85 per cent of people thought there should be greater control over the way fast foods are promoted to children. But there's no getting away from the fact that we also influence the way our kids think and act – and that includes the food choices they make. In fact, the Health Development Agency says parents are the key to tackling children's obesity, and that involving both parents and children together is the best way forward.

Parents think that, too – nine out of ten people think parents bear the main responsibility for shaping eating and exercise habits. Researchers at Exeter University found that children who perceive they have an active mother are more likely to be active themselves. When it comes to food, **if kids see adults at home eating a diet low in healthy options and high in fatty, sugary meals and snacks, they are likely to think this is normal**. One study, published in 2003 in the journal *Health Psychology*, found that parents give their children fatty and sugary foods to calm them down when they're stressed, and that children copy their parents and reach for these foods when they're under pressure from things like school worries or family troubles.

For many parents, though, eating this way is the norm. If they've always eaten like this, they might not know it's unhealthy. Many parents have trouble understanding that there could be a problem with their child's eating habits and weight in the first place. In one study, 40 per cent of parents of obese children didn't think their kids had a weight problem, and a third of obese girls and half of obese boys were described as 'about right' by their mums. Nicki says, 'It can be hard to understand how to improve your children's diet, and even harder to get them to make healthy choices. But through Inch Loss Kids, I've seen the misery being overweight can cause children and the difference shifting those pounds can make to how they feel about themselves.'

Inactivity

Our kids are becoming less and less active as time goes by. Researchers have found that children are so inactive even some three-year-olds can be classed as couch potatoes. Experts recommend that children aged three to five should have at least an hour of moderate to vigorous exercise a day. But researchers found that children of this age were typically active for only 20–25 minutes. Some pre-school kids actually get so little exercise they spend a frightening 80 per cent of their week being inactive.

And the picture isn't much better for older children. One study found that children aged 5–11 spend an average of 5.7 hours each weekend watching television, 3.8 hours with friends and 3.1 hours on the computer. In comparison, they spent a total of 4 hours on physical activity. Kids in the 11–16 age group spent 9.9 hours on the computer or watching television and just 3.8 hours on physical activity. One UK study of 10–13-year-olds found that most fell short of the Department of Health's recommended energy expenditure. At weekends, some were so inactive that their activity levels were the same as bed-ridden hospital patients. One girl spent the day in bed, eating, watching television and playing video games, only getting up to use the toilet. When you consider that weight gain occurs when input (food) is greater than output (activity), it's easy to see how being less active is affecting our kids.

'SO WHAT?'

You might well say to yourself, 'What does all of this matter?' Well, eating the wrong foods and being inactive can increase the risk of overweight and obesity, and with it both physical and emotional problems. We're talking about your children's future here – do you really want these problems to be a part of their lives?

Physical Problems

Figures show that obese teenagers have a 70 per cent chance of becoming overweight or obese adults (80 per cent if one or more parent is overweight or obese). Health problems that come with being obese include:

- **Type 2 diabetes**. This always used to be thought of as an adults' disease. However, it has recently been detected in some UK children between the ages of 13 and 15. Youngsters who develop this form of diabetes have an increased risk of heart, eye and kidney diseases.
- **Hyperlipidaemia.** This is raised levels of fat in the blood – the most commonly heard of is cholesterol

but others include triglycerides and lipoproteins. Obese children tend to have higher levels of 'bad' cholesterol and lower levels of 'good' cholesterol, a pattern that's strongly associated with heart disease in adulthood.
- **Raised blood pressure.** Obese children and teenagers are nine times more likely to have raised blood pressure than children of normal weight. If it's untreated, it can lead to stroke, heart disease and kidney problems.
- **Breathing difficulties.** Obesity in children is a significant risk factor for coughing and wheezing. Other research suggests that overweight children are 77 per cent more likely to have asthma than other children.
- **Sleep apnoea.** This is a condition where you stop breathing for periods of up to 10 seconds while you're asleep, and it affects seven per cent of obese children. It can stop a child getting a good night's sleep, which in turn can affect such factors as concentration levels at school.

Emotional Problems

It's not just extra pounds that overweight or obese children carry around with them – they also shoulder psychological burdens. These children are more likely to suffer from low self-esteem caused by teasing and bullying. In fact, research has discovered that the parents

Young Sugar Addicts

of obese children take them on holiday more, change their school or even move house to protect them from teasing and bullying by other children. It's a sad fact, but studies also suggest that people assume overweight people are lazy, unclean and don't have feelings. So what can you do about it? In the next chapter, we're going to show you how you can help kids to get on the path to a healthier lifestyle. The chapter also contains advice for older kids on how to make these changes themselves.

6
Helping Young Sugar Addicts

As we saw in the previous chapter, a sugary diet is bad news for our kids, setting them on the road to excess weight gain and all the problems that brings with it. This is something that has been addressed by Nicki and her GMTV colleagues – including clinical psychologist Dr Paul Chadwick of charity Weight Concern – as part of Inch Loss Juniors. In this chapter, Nicki shares some of the tips that have helped so many teenagers aged 13–15 take on a healthier way of life – without feeling they're 'odd' or missing out on what their friends do.

HOW THIS BOOK CAN HELP KIDS – AND PARENTS!
Faddy diets are just as bad for kids as they are for adults – discouraging sensible, healthy eating and often putting the body in 'starvation mode', which helps it to store fat. As children keep growing until they are at least 19, we're not recommending that they go through the 21 days of the Sugar Addicts' Diet. But they can eat the foods recommended in the Diet, including the sugar substitutes. After all, these are nutritious, healthy foods

SUGAR ADDICTS' DIET

that are just as good for children as they are for adults.

The philosophy of the Sugar Addicts' Diet is a healthy way of life, not a faddy diet that suggests you eat peculiar or even dangerous foods. The philosophy of eating carbs with protein, having good snacks and incorporating exercise into your daily routine are all sensible concepts that will help kids stay the right size for their age. Many of the nutrients in these foods, such as omega 3 oils, are vital for brain function, so they can help kids stay alert and perform well at school. Incorporating these steps into their lifestyle will also give them more energy – all of which adds up to happy kids.

Important

We're not recommending that you put your children on a diet – that can only be a decision for you and your child under medical supervision. But some of the tips we are offering here may help you understand how to incorporate healthy eating and exercise into your family's life to get them on the path to being healthier.

KEEPING A FOOD DIARY

As we said in Chapter 3, keeping a food diary can be a real help when it comes to understanding what you eat, why you eat it and when you choose to do it. It's the same for kids – if you write down what you're eating, you can keep track of it and you'll know where changes need to be made.

Action

Kids: At the end of each day – for example, when you're watching television or finishing your homework – write down what you've eaten that day. You could do it once a week but it's very likely you'll forget what you've eaten. At the end of the week, take a look at your diary and see what foods or drinks are in there, then compare it to the lists of 'Foods you can eat', 'Occasional treats' and 'Foods to avoid' in Chapter 8. Ask your parents to do this with you. Ideally, if you're eating healthily you'll have more foods from the first list than the second two. If there are more from the second two, you know there's room for some improvement.

Remember: This isn't about losing weight. It's about trying to eat healthier foods and getting a bit more active.

Nicki's Tips

Keeping a food diary will help you show your parents how well you've done, which is vital for earning your rewards (see 'Planning Rewards' on page 104).

Parents: If you're following the Sugar Addicts' Diet yourself, you could fill in your food diary with your child. If you're not, follow the diary suggestions at the end of Chapter 3. Although adults are asked to write down how they feel at certain times of the day, don't get kids to do this. The last thing we want is for them to start associating food with feelings, as this can lead to unhealthy, obsessive attitudes towards food. Just get them to fill in what they're eating and how much exercise they're getting. Take a look at the diary at the end of each day and work out, from the lists in Chapter 8, where there could be room for improvement.

SETTING GOALS

Having goals is really important for motivation. It can help you to focus on what you have to achieve without losing interest or faith in yourself. On Inch Loss Juniors, Nicki and clinical psychologist Dr Paul Chadwick recommended having '**SMART**' goals – **S**pecific, **M**easurable, **A**chievable, **R**elevant and **T**ime-limited. Here's what they mean:

Specific: Goals should be something like 'reduce the number of fizzy drinks each week' rather than 'be more healthy' or 'eat less'. Those are far too 'fuzzy' to mean anything.
Measurable: Goals should be something you can measure. A good example would be 'ride my bike' or

'eat fewer crisps'. A better goal would be 'ride my bike for 20 minutes twice a week' or 'eat just two packets of crisps per week'.
Achievable: It's easy to be over-ambitious when it comes to setting goals. But that could play against you and you could end up just feeling bad about yourself. A good goal might be 'walk to school instead of getting a lift' rather than 'go for a run seven times a week'.
Relevant: When you're setting your goal, you need to ask, 'Does this really apply to my life?' For example, a bad goal would be to say 'give up doughnuts' when you know you only eat them every few months, but a good goal would be 'have chocolate twice a week instead of twice a day'.
Time-limited: Put time 'markers' on your goals. So instead of saying to yourself 'go swimming', say 'go swimming twice by next Tuesday'.

Action
Kids: Start with small achievable goals – writing day one of your food diary is a brilliant first goal. You can then work up to more difficult ones as time goes by.

Remember: Don't give up or be angry with yourself if you don't achieve a goal. It could be it was too difficult, so go for a less difficult goal and start again. Don't forget to reward yourself. This isn't meant to be punishment!

Parents: Make sure you are prepared to help your child reach their goals. Make sure you discuss their goals with them. After all, you are a key part of their success. If one of their goals is to drink fewer fizzy drinks, then having delicious alternatives for them in the fridge or cupboard will help them achieve it.

EATING PROPERLY

Eating properly is about the food you eat and *how* you eat it. Eating regularly helps to establish a routine so you ensure you get the intake of nutrients you need. The Sugar Addicts' Diet aims to help adults eat properly and regularly to help stabilize blood-sugar levels. Kids need steady blood-sugar levels, too, and eating routines can help achieve this.

Action

Kids: It's so easy to munch away without even thinking about it. Whether we're sitting watching telly or playing a computer game, we can find we've eaten our way through a whole packet of sweets or biscuits without even really tasting them. Here's something for you to have a go at:

- **Try eating without distractions**. Don't eat while you're watching telly, doing homework or walking down the road with friends.

- **Sit down and eat**. Only eat when you're sitting down with the purpose of eating, such as at the dinner table or in a restaurant. This will soon help you to stop 'aimless' eating.
- **Eat slowly**. Tempted to gulp your food down? Make sure you put your knife and fork down between each mouthful. You'll be surprised at how that slows things down! If you're eating with your hands, make sure you chew well and swallow your mouthful before taking the next one rather than eating like a conveyor belt!

Parents:
- **Make sure kids have breakfast**. Breakfast helps to raise blood-sugar levels that have dropped overnight and will help kids function more effectively. Evidence also suggests academic performance can be boosted by a high-energy breakfast. See Chapter 9 for breakfast ideas. Do they say they haven't got time for breakfast? Get them up earlier!
- **Get them to eat regularly and have healthy snacks**. Eat with them, or at least make sure one parent or family member eats with them to make it more of an 'occasion'. Have healthy snacks rather than sugary, fatty ones ready in the fridge or cupboard. Look at the snack options in Chapter 9 for some ideas.

- **Eat a 'proper' meal at lunchtime.** This should either be a healthy packed lunch or getting your kid to agree to a school meal rather than a fast-food option.
- **Reduce portion sizes.** As a parent, it's you who doles out the food at the dinner table. If you're facing resistance as you try and make the portion sizes smaller, choose smaller plates for all the family so that no one feels singled out for special treatment.

GETTING MORE ACTIVE

Ask most kids about activity and they'll probably groan and say, 'We do PE at school.' But activity levels are more than about timetabled exercise – they're about general activity levels, too.

Action

Kids: If someone says 'exercise' to you, your heart may well sink as you think about doing sports you don't like and getting hot and sweaty. Well, here are some tips that we hope won't feel like punishment. Nicki says, 'The key to getting more active is to slowly increase your activity levels, rather than going from no activity to high activity. Even walking or cycling to the newsagent rather than getting your mum to give you a lift is a step in the right direction.'

- **Frisbee.** Don't worry if you have no co-ordination and you throw or catch badly. The worse you are, the

Helping Young Sugar Addicts

better the workout will be because you'll spend half your time running to pick up missed Frisbees! It's a great game to improve both fitness and co-ordination and burns up 250 calories per hour. If you get good, you can even take it up competitively with Ultimate Frisbee. Find out more at www.ukultimate.com

- **Walk the dog**. Sounds so simple but power-walking the dog for half an hour can burn up 200–300 calories. If you head for the hills, your muscles have to work harder because you're working against gravity.
- **Baby-sit**. Offer to baby-sit and you can take the children outside or to the park to play. Letting them run you ragged is a great way of getting exercise – and it'll be earning you money in the process.
- **Do your chores**. Sounds dull? You'll please your mum and you'll also get some exercise in the process. See if your parents will give you some money to do more around the house, whether it's vacuuming, polishing or washing the car.
- **Get some skates**. Burn 570 calories an hour roller skating. Once you've mastered the basics, increase the intensity by including some hills, varying your pace and adding strength moves, such as the 'swizzle' (let your legs travel apart, then squeeze your inner thighs to draw them together). Research shows that inline skating works some lower body muscles (particularly the thighs) better than running – and it'll improve your balance and core stability too.

SUGAR ADDICTS' DIET

Parents:
- **Organize a picnic**. If the weather's nice, get a healthy picnic together and go to your local park, armed with plenty of games to play such as Frisbee, rounders or badminton.
- **Row a boat**. Maybe you can incorporate this into your picnic! Rowing a real boat with the kids can be a laugh and give you all a great buzz. Once you're proficient, you can burn 250–350 calories per half hour. You'll also strengthen and tone your legs, back and arms. Want to know more? Find a club at www.ara-rowing.org
- **Buy a bike**. Cycling can burn 150–360 calories an hour. It's not just the gradients that increase your energy expenditure – when you rock the bike from side to side to get up a steep slope or 'loft' (pull up the handlebars to get the front wheel over obstacles in the path), you work your upper body muscles too. Make sure you and the kids wear helmets and reflector vests, and have the saddle adjusted correctly. As you sit, your knee should be slightly bent on the down stroke. The proper cycling action is a complete circle, pushing down for the first half of the stroke and pulling up with the second, using every muscle in your legs. No excuses – get on your bikes!
- **Do some gardening**. We're not suggesting you turn into Charlie Dimmock but even a little pottering around in the garden can get the heart rate going and

Helping Young Sugar Addicts

burn up calories. Gardening (from planting, watering and weeding to mowing the lawn) can burn 120–330 calories an hour. The main benefit of gardening is the cumulative effect of carrying, bending, stooping, twisting and digging for the whole body. Carrying garden moss for instance, uses more muscles and burns more calories than standing and watering. Give younger children their own plants to tend to get them interested (sunflowers are good – have a 'whose sunflower is tallest' competition).

- **Walk the dog together**. If the dog-walking has become your responsibility, try sharing it by suggesting you walk him together each evening before or after your meal. While you're walking, don't just stand at one end of a field and throw the ball. Walk round with the dog so that it's not just him who gets the exercise.
- **Play childhood games**. Don't just watch them play – join in with them! Choose leapfrog or hopscotch, then add 'bounce' to increase calorie expenditure by 10 per cent. Draw an imaginary cross on the ground, stand in the top left-hand square and jump right, back, left, then forward. Continue for 30 seconds. Rest for 30 seconds and repeat twice. Or try skipping – it's a great fun, do-anywhere exercise and can burn 300–450 calories an hour.

PLANNING REWARDS

We all need rewards for doing things we perhaps don't want to do. Without rewards or incentives, we soon lose interest and ditch our good intentions. This also applies to trying to cultivate a healthier lifestyle – there's got to be something to make it interesting when the competition from junk food and inactivity is so great! Well, here's how you can do it.

Action
Kids:
- **Get something you want**. A reward has to be something you want or it's not a reward at all. Be realistic, though – asking for a pet rat when your mum has a phobia of them might not be met with much enthusiasm!
- **Rewards should equal achievements**. You know when you've tried hard and you know when you haven't – come on, we all do! So if you haven't put that much effort into changing your habits, then don't expect a big reward for it. Remember – small achievements earn you small rewards while big achievements get bigger rewards. Keep that in mind and it could really help you try that little bit harder.
- **Keep writing your food diary**. As well as enabling you to keep track of what you're eating and how much you're exercising, your diary can also act as proof of how you deserve your rewards!

Helping Young Sugar Addicts

Parents:

- **Don't reward weight loss.** Kids go through phases when they'll put on weight because they're having a growth spurt, so measuring weight may not be representative of how healthy they are. A better approach is to focus on rewarding healthy habits, such as them eating more fruit.
- **Don't talk negatively about food.** It's important to take a keen interest in what your child is eating, especially if you feel they're scoffing too much junk. But there's a fine line between concern and obsession, and if you start talking negatively about food or talking about food every time something passes their lips, you could end up in real trouble. Always see the positive in what they've done rather than focusing onhow they could have done it better.
- **Small rewards are better than big ones.** Telling kids they can have something small each week (like a new football or a magazine) is better for motivation than a big reward they have to wait for, such as a trip abroad in the summer.
- **Don't use food to reward.** Using food as a reward for good behaviour or punishment for bad is putting an unhealthy focus on food. It should be viewed as sustenance – a way of satisfying hunger – not as emotional currency. Don't do it yourself and get other people who may be using food as 'treats'

(such as relatives) to stop doing it, too. There are plenty of other types of rewards available to you.

TIPS FOR PARENTS

- **Don't be a 'bossy adult'.** Kids feel like adults spend the whole time bossing them around anyway, and most of the time it makes them shut off and ignore you. Being bossy about them eating the right foods or exercising isn't the right approach. You're much more likely to make an impression if you encourage, reward and are a good role model yourself (kids hate hypocrites!).
- **Be a good role model.** There's nothing worse than eating healthily while someone at the table is gorging on a delicious but fatty pizza or a burger with all the trimmings. It does nothing for motivation. Most of us can benefit from improving our lifestyle a little, from eating more healthily to getting off our backsides and moving more. Make sure you do these things, too; don't just say them.
- **Listen to their ideas.** A healthier lifestyle doesn't have to be a one-way street. Children can be the source of many bright ideas about a healthier lifestyle, often picked up from friends or in lessons. Also, if it's their health you're concerned about, it's important that they feel involved and empowered by the process of getting healthier. Being healthy shouldn't be something imposed upon them but

something they can feel in charge of. Family meetings to discuss activities or meals for the week are a good way to help everyone feel involved.
- **Be a smart shopper**. Shopping for the 'right' foods is a chore in itself – supermarkets are full of tempting but unhealthy foods that are hard to resist. Beware of foods that are marketed towards children, such as packaging with cartoon figures or 'shaped' foods. Many of these are high in sugar and fat, not to mention additives and colourings. Use our list of sugars in Chapter 8 to help you locate added sugars in the foods you're buying.
- **Shop without them!** The lure of foods advertised by celebrities, special on-pack promotions and free gifts can often be too much for children to resist. And you may well buy these foods just to shut them up! To avoid 'pester power', do the big supermarket shop without the kids, or try it online through one of the big supermarkets. That way you won't find yourself giving in to them when they say, 'Oh mum, can't we try this …'
- **… Or enlist their help**. For example, when you're being a 'sugar detective', get kids involved, too, by making a game out of reading labels. It'll also help them understand what's in food and what they're eating.
- **Make food interesting**. Lure them away from those unhealthy choices by discovering how

interesting healthy food can actually be. Most of us wouldn't know how to use a recipe book if it fell out of the sky and hit us on the head, but it doesn't have to be difficult. Try some of the recipes in Chapter 15 as a good starting point.
- **Get active**. We don't just mean getting out of the armchair (though you really ought to be doing that, too!). We're also talking about getting your voice heard as a parent. The Food Commission set up The Parents' Jury in March 2002 to help parents voice their concern about the quality of children's food and the ways it is marketed (such as through celebrities or the placing of sweets at checkouts). All parents of children aged 2–16 are welcome to take part. Visit www.parentsjury.org for further information or to find out how to join the jury.
- **Prevent them developing a sweet tooth**. As we saw in Chapter 1, it's possible to steer young children in the direction of a high-sugar diet by feeding their natural desire – but the good news is you can also help prevent this happening. If your kids are older and already love sugar, you'll hopefully find that some of the tips outlined above will help you make changes to their diet and lifestyle to stop sugar being so influential. What about if your kids are younger? Professor Aubrey Sheihan says, 'Don't deny them sugary foods when they are weaning but try to limit them.' Try to keep the sweetness 'threshold' low by

offering naturally sweet foods such as fruit rather than intensely sweetened foods such as chocolate, cakes or sweets. If you want to give them these foods, make them small, occasional treats. Try and retrain the palate of older kids by adopting the same tactic.

HOW SCHOOLS CAN HELP

It's not only parents who are responsible for helping kids achieve a healthier, more active lifestyle. As we saw in the last chapter, many different people and organizations play their part. School also has a role to play. The Food Standards Agency's Action Plan is a series of proposals aimed at tackling factors affecting children's poor diets, such as advertising. But it's also planning to work with schools to make healthier foods a priority, such as by targeting vending machines to increase the range of healthy options.

This kind of pressure can come from you, too. As a parent, you have the right to voice your opinion to the school about how they're running things – and that doesn't just mean as far as lessons are concerned. If you want to make a difference and help your kid now and in the future, here are some suggestions you as parents can make to help turn you child's school into a healthier place:

- **Green vending machines**. A huge 79 per cent of parents would like to see a ban on vending machines offering pupils unhealthy options. They have a right to be concerned – surveys show that almost 7 out of 10 children eat at least one packet of crisps most days of the week, while more than one in three eats chocolate each day. But there is an alternative. Companies including Absolute Vending will install healthy vending machines into schools to provide fruit juices, potato-crisp alternatives and dried fruit pieces. Your school will be able to look into this for you.

- **Offering interesting healthy food**. School-meal services tend to be contracted out which generally means the provider who offers the cheapest deal wins the contract. Cheap food tends to be high in fat and sugar so that's what ends up on our kids' plates. If your kids are going to have a school meal, you'll want to be sure it's balanced and healthy. Healthy food doesn't have to be dull – speak to your school about how they can influence the meal provider to offer your kids something that's nourishing as well as interesting to eat.
- **Get into H_2O**. Surveys show that 20 per cent of kids – that's one in five – have more than four cans of pop a day. One MP, Jon Owen Jones, is trying to get a bill through Parliament banning vending machines offering these drinks, and his proposals are being backed by organizations including the British Heart Foundation. Bowing to parental pressure, Coca-Cola has been persuaded to remove its logos from the 4,000 machines it operates in UK schools. One thing you

could suggest as a parent is that your school installs water coolers to give kids something healthier to drink. More and more schools are doing this – make yours one of them.
- **Breakfast Club**. Figures show that 17 per cent of children leave home each morning without eating breakfast. Starting the day hungry can affect concentration and leave kids more open to choosing junk-food options through the day. The government's Breakfast Club initiative aims to help make breakfast a part of kids' everyday lives. Your school could start up a Breakfast Club. For further information, visit www.breakfast-club.co.uk. But make sure you lobby your school for healthy options in the club – one study found that many clubs fail to offer fruit or cereals and give pupils unhealthy choices such as doughnuts and crisps instead.
- **Suggest different activity options**. If your own memories of sports at school are of windy cross-country runs or freezing showers, then it may be hard for you to be enthusiastic about school sports to your kids. But kids can have a positive experience if they're taking part in something they can really get into. If the school is not already offering it, why not suggest they have classes in such activities as aerobics or salsa. In other words, something that will appeal to kids.
- **Contact your local MP**. It sounds like a scary thing to do and you may well say, 'What's the point? I can't

make a difference.' But there are plenty of examples where 'people power' has done exactly that. How about this to get you wound up – despite rising child-obesity rates, many local authorities continue to sell off playing fields at a rate of one every three weeks. Figures show that 113 playing fields were sold off between 1996 and 2002 – an average of 19 a year. If no one ever declares actions like this unacceptable, they keep on happening. Want to know how to get in contact with your local MP? Find a directory of MPs at www.parliament.uk

7
Where Sugar is Lurking

In most food categories, you'll find examples that are low in sugar and those that are high. Some will strike you as more obvious than others – for example, it'd be no surprise to find sugar in sweets or chocolate. But others may surprise you. They certainly came as a shock to us.

Below is a list of some food categories where we found examples that contained sugar. Remember – not all of the foods in these categories contain sugar. Many plain cottage cheeses, for example, are sugar-free. What we're trying to show you is that **sugar can lurk in the most unexpected places**. And, of course, this isn't an exhaustive list – there are millions of products out there. The key for you is to understand this and to realize that the only way to be sure about what you're eating is to check the label before you buy it.

Dips – e.g. Sainsbury's fresh onion and garlic dip, Sainsbury's fresh guacamole dip, taramasalata, Tesco vine-ripened tomato salsa, Tesco reduced-fat sour cream and chive dip, Tesco selection dip multipack, Walkers Doritos Dippas, Pataks raita dip

Cottage cheese – e.g. Sainsbury's chargrilled vegetables cottage cheese, Sainsbury's Be Good To Yourself prawn cocktail cottage cheese & coronation chicken cottage cheese, Tesco Healthy Living tuna and sweetcorn cottage cheese

Sandwich meats – e.g. Bernard Matthews premium Norfolk turkey breast, Tesco wafer-thin beef, Tesco smoked ham, Tesco American-style pastrami, Sainsbury's wafer-thin chicken

Drinking yoghurts with beneficial bacteria – e.g. Benecol drinking yoghurt, Danone Actimel

Crisps and snacks – This is the area that surprised us the most. Many snacks such as onion rings or cheese puffs contain sugar in one form or another. Examples: Sainsbury's cheese savouries, Sainsbury's onion ring snacks, Golden Wonder wheat crunchies, Nice 'n' Spicy Nik Naks (contain saccharine), Walkers cheese and onion crisps, Walkers pickled onion Monster Munch, Sharwood's prawn crackers, Golden Wonder salt and vinegar flavour crunchy fries, Pringles potato snacks (sour cream and onion, plus many other flavours), Sainsbury's luxury hickory smoke coated nuts, Sainsbury's dry roasted peanuts, Walker's Thai Sweet Chilli Sensations, Kellogg's Special K Lite Bites (sun-dried tomato, tikka and cheese flavours), Tesco pickled onion Beast Snacks

'Healthier' products – e.g. Sainsbury's Be Good To Yourself digestive biscuits, custard creams, milk chocolate digestives (they say they contain 25 per cent less fat but they're packed with sugar), Weight Watchers' real chocolate-chip cookies, Tesco Healthy Living American chicken fajitas, Healthy Fox's Officially Low Fat Apple Crumble Cookies, Tesco Healthy Living cranberry and blackcurrant cereal bars
Sauces and condiments – e.g. tomato ketchup (Heinz, Daddies, Tesco), some mayonnaise (e.g. Sainsbury's Be Good To Yourself thick and creamy mayonnaise), HP Brown Sauce, HP Fruity Sauce, Tesco fruity sauce, Amoy light soy sauce
Kids' lunch box and other foods – e.g. Dairylea Dunkers Jumbo Munch, Dairylea Lunchables Tender Turkey, Dairylea Stack 'Ems, Dairylea hotdogs, Attack a Snack chicken wrap, Tesco Kids 15 mini hotdogs, Fruit Bowl school bars ('ideal for lunchboxes'), Ribena Light juice drink, Ribena blackcurrant juice drink (packaging says it's rich in vitamin C and contains real fruit juice but it also contains glucose, fructose syrup and sucrose), Sainsbury's Blue Parrot Café apple and blackcurrant juice drink, Heinz pasta shapes (e.g. Teletubbies, Tweenies, Thomas the Tank Engine), HP pasta shapes (Bob the Builder, Loony Tunes, Action Man), Bernard Matthews Norfolk Dinosaur Turkey Roll, Pepperami
Potato products – e.g. Sainsbury's Occasions spicy potato wedges, McCain savoury potato wedges (nicely

spiced), Sainsbury's American-style oven chips, Pom-Bear original teddy-shaped snacks
Cooking sauces – e.g. Knorr Chicken Tonight country French sauce, Knorr ragu sauce (spicy, traditional and original varieties), Loyd Grossman's tomato and basil pasta sauce, Sharwood's medium dhansak sauce, Ragu Bolognaise sauce, Patak's mild korma sauce, Old El Paso fajita cooking sauce, Tesco Healthy Living sweet and sour cooking sauce

---

Nicki's Tips

Look out for the words 'coated', 'smoked' or 'flavoured' when you're buying foods. In my experience, this often means they contain sugar in some form (e.g. lactose or maltodextrin). Check the ingredients before you buy. Look at the list of sugar and the different names it goes by in Chapter 8. This way you'll know what to look for when reading labels in the supermarket.

Part 2:

The Sugar Addict's Tools for Recovery

8
What to Eat

We tackle this first because in order to make any headway – and before you even think about giving up sugar – you've got to stabilize what you're eating and get blood-sugar levels under control. If you don't feel hungry, you'll feel physically better and more mentally alert – and far more capable of making positive decisions about what you eat, rather than reaching for the biscuit tin.

This is the basis for being able to give up sugar – don't see it as dull or unnecessary. If you can master this part of the plan and stick with it, then when you actually give up sugar you won't feel like someone's knocked you for six. Don't start to take foods out of your diet yet – we'll be advising you on when to do that once you start the plan. Here is the list of actions you'll be incorporating into your 21-day plan:

1 Foods you can eat
2. Occasional treats
3. Foods to avoid
4. Recognizing sugars

5. Drink more liquids
6. Eat the 'right fats'

FOODS YOU CAN EAT

This list will help you pick foods that won't give you an empty 'rush'. It includes good carbohydrates (found in wholemeal produce and vegetables such as cabbage and tomatoes) and protein (including animal protein such as meat and eggs and vegetable protein such as Quorn or kidney beans).

The Glycaemic Index (GI) (see page 40) ranks foods from 1 to 100, according to how quickly they cause your blood-glucose levels to rise. The higher the number, the quicker the food causes a rise in levels. So, for example, sugar has a high GI while wholemeal foods tend to be lower on the scale. If you're trying to level out your blood sugar to knock sugar cravings on the head, the last thing you want is lots of insulin in your blood followed by a sugar dip. Low GI is the key – you don't need to know exactly what these foods are but you'll find that the carbohydrates we recommend in the Sugar Addicts' Diet are low GI. And where we identify or suggest a food that's higher GI, we explain why and how to eat it to minimize the effect on your blood-glucose levels. The list below provides plenty of information for you about what you can eat on the 21-day plan.

What to Eat

Complex Carbohydrates

- **'Grainy' bread**. Bread is full of contradictions when it comes to GI. It turns out that wholemeal (i.e. brown but without whole seeds in it) has a GI only marginally lower than white bread. But a good rule of thumb here is that the grainier the bread, the better it is for GI. The 'bits' in it (grains, nuts and seeds) help to reduce the speed at which the carbohydrates break down, which is a good thing. Include more grainy varieties in your diet, and even sourdough bread, which has a low GI. Examples include Vogel's, Burgen or simple granary bread.
- **Whole-grain cereal** (e.g. porridge oats, Nestlé Shredded Wheat. See breakfast options in Chapter 9).
- **Pasta**. All pasta, whether white or wholemeal, has a low GI (white spaghetti has a GI of 41, wholemeal has a GI of 37). It's still good to try brown pasta as this should help to develop your task for healthier 'brown' foods. Whatever your choice, try to eat it 'al dente' (slightly hard) rather than overcooked and soft as this increases its GI. There's some evidence to suggest 'thicker' pasta has a lower GI than 'thinner' (e.g. fettuccini is better than spaghetti).
- **Potatoes with their skins**. Whether it's jacket potato, new potatoes, potato wedges or mashed potatoes, they're fine in moderation as long as they have their skins and you combine them with protein and other vegetables. The best way to eat baked potatoes is to

select two or three smaller ones rather than one big one so you have a greater ratio of skin to potato. Baby new potatoes are also a good, low-GI way to eat potatoes.
- **Sweet potatoes**. These are a good alternative to normal potatoes as they have a lower GI.
- **Basmati rice**. Unlike other varieties of white rice, basmati (commonly used in southern Asian cuisine such as Indian) has a low GI so is fine to eat.
- **Brown rice** (e.g. American whole-grain, brown basmati or wild rice, Sainsbury's boil-in-the-bag brown rice, Uncle Ben's whole-grain rice).
- **Noodles**. These are low GI, but steer clear of flavoured instant noodles as these are high in other ingredients such as additives and bad fats (some instant noodles have up to 20g of fat in each container). Choose egg noodles instead.
- **Corn tortillas**. Choose these rather than the wheat variety.
- **Taco shells**.
- **Unsweetened/unsalted popcorn**.

Fresh Produce

Fruit and vegetables are, in fact, carbohydrates. It's important to bear this in mind when you're trying to combine protein with complex carbs (as we'll be discussing in Chapter 9). They are also high in fibre, which you need for a steady carbohydrate breakdown (as opposed to fast breakdown which can lead to a sugar 'high').

Although we're advised to eat five portions of fruit and veg a day, it's important to remember that some fruit and veg are more 'stabilizing' for your blood-sugar levels than others. In fact, some fruits are so naturally high in sugar and low in fibre that they are more like refined carbohydrates (or the 'sneaky' sugars we talked about in Chapter 3). These break down quickly in the body rather than at a slow, even rate. On the Sugar Addicts' Diet you are allowed to eat high and medium GI fruit and veg, but be aware that you're better off choosing from the low GI lists. Here's the low-down on what you can eat:

- **Vegetables** – especially low GI ones:
  Low GI veg: leeks, onions, broccoli, cauliflower, cabbage, spinach, asparagus, peppers, lettuce, tomatoes, mushrooms, bean sprouts.
  Medium GI veg: carrots, turnips, courgettes, pumpkin, beetroot, avocados.
  High GI veg: potatoes, sweet potatoes, parsnips, peas, aubergines.

Of your five portions of fruit and veg a day, try to make three or more of them low to medium GI vegetables.

SUGAR ADDICTS' DIET

- **Fruit** (fresh, baked, canned in fruit juice rather than syrup, or stewed but without added sugar) – especially low GI ones:
  Low GI fruit: blueberries, blackberries, cherries, grapefruit, raspberries, strawberries.
  Medium GI fruit: peaches, pineapples, mangoes, papayas, olives.
  High GI fruit: bananas, dates, figs, grapes, prunes, raisins and watermelon. Dried fruit and fruit juices also have a high GI.

Of your five portions of fruit and veg a day, make fruit no more than two of them.

Nicki's Tips

Not all fruit and veg are equal! As a general rule of thumb, the high GI ones act like carbs so always make sure you eat them with some protein.

Protein

Whether in plant or animal form, protein foods trigger the release of a hormone that tells us we're no longer hungry. Foods rich in protein have also been shown to keep us feeling fuller for longer. If proteins are included in our meals and snacks, we're less likely to be struck by the kind of hunger that gets us reaching for a sugary lift in the middle of the afternoon.

What to Eat

Animal
- **Lean meat** (e.g. turkey and chicken, lean beef).
- **Eggs** (especially Columbus eggs containing Omega-3 oils).
- **Fish**, especially oily fish (e.g. mackerel, halibut, tuna and salmon).
- **Low-fat dairy produce**, including semi-skimmed/skimmed milk, low-fat cheese, cottage cheese (including varieties with chives or pineapple) and plain yoghurt.

Vegetable
- **Vegetarian meat alternatives** (e.g. tofu and Quorn).
- **Nuts and seeds** (e.g. unsalted almonds, walnuts, Brazil nuts, sunflower seeds, pumpkin seeds).
- **Pulses and lentils** (e.g. red kidney beans, chickpeas, soya beans, Heinz Curried Beans with no added sugar, Sainsbury's Organic Baked Beans).
- **Houmous** (a dip made from chickpeas and sesame-based tahini).

Occasional Treats

Why: As well as trying to even out the highs and lows produced by sugar, we're also trying to get rid of your craving for sweet tastes. You may never get over this if you're constantly exposing yourself to sweet foods, and this includes sugar substitutes. They don't cause insulin to be released so they could be a solution if you're in need of a 'stepping stone' to a sugar-free diet, or as an occasional sweet treat once you've ditched the sugar. As for honey and molasses, don't be fooled into thinking they're not sugar because they are. If you're really trying to do this properly, don't eat them. They still give a sugar rush.

- **Artificially sweetened products**. 'Low-sugar' or diabetic products (e.g. Boots no added sugar fruit gums, Thorntons diabetic chocolate assortment), foods containing sweeteners such as Splenda, saccharine or NutraSweet (e.g. Diet Coke). See the list of sweeteners below. Visit www.sugarfreesuperstore.co.uk
- **Honey**. It's still sugar, but if you have to have a dab of sugar then make it honey – preferably manuka honey from New Zealand which has all kinds of health benefits as well as being delicious. Watch out as many commercial brands of honey have sugar added to them. Why, we don't know – we think it's sweet enough as it is!
- **Molasses**. This is still a sugar, but it's unrefined and contains at least some nutrients, namely potassium, calcium, magnesium, iron, copper and manganese, all of which your body uses for vital functions, such as metabolism.
- **Alcohol**. This is a stimulant, like tea and coffee (see below). Women should restrict their intake to a maximum of 14 units a week (a unit being a small

glass of 8 per cent proof wine). Remember – this is a maximum, not a goal to work towards! Wondering what drink to go for? Avoid alcopops as they are loaded with sugar. Beer contains high levels of maltose (a sugar) which heads straight for the bloodstream. Opt instead for wine (best is a dry white wine spritzer with fizzy water or soda, not lemonade) or vodka, which is a pure alcohol (again, with fizzy water, soda or a small amount of pure fruit juice). Don't use tonic water as a mixer as it contains sugar (the slimline version contains sweeteners).

- **All the foods in the 'avoid' list!** You're only human – if you succumb to these foods once in a while, don't feel bad about it. The aim is to try and get to a position where you can occasionally eat them without bingeing or falling off the wagon.
- **Processed meats**. Avoid fatty meats and meat products, such as salamis, sausages and meat pies, or any meat with visible fat or rind such as pork chops. These should be eaten only occasionally as they are high in saturated fats, a high intake of which can increase the risk of conditions such as heart disease.
- **Full fat dairy produce** (including hard cheese, full-fat cottage cheese and yoghurt). Again, these are high in saturated fats (the 'wrong' type of fats). People sometimes say, 'You never see a fat vegetarian.' Wrong! You do if they substitute meat with full-fat dairy products and eat cheese at every meal. Low-fat

SUGAR ADDICTS' DIET

cheeses such as Edam or Philadelphia Light are just as tasty and a great choice for the daily two to three portions of dairy produce we recommend.
- **Tea and coffee.** You may wonder why you have to cut down on these things. Like sugar and alcohol, tea and coffee are stimulants, and the more of a stimulant you have, the more you crave it. If you're already addicted to sugar, you're trying to get your body away from craving it – and craving other addictive things. But we're not saying you can't have that cuppa to get you going in the morning – just have it with your protein and carb breakfast or mid-morning snack. For substitutes, see 'Drink more liquids' on page 134.

FOODS TO AVOID
Why: These are the kinds of food you often reach for when you're in need of a sugar 'fix'. However, shortly after you've satisfied the craving, you feel low in energy and in need of yet another sugar and refined carb boost. This list includes sugars and quick-release (refined) carbohydrates that can give you a high followed by a dip.

Refined/'Sneaky' Sugars
- White bread (including rolls, white pitta bread)
- White bagels
- Croissants
- Doughnuts
- Cakes

What to Eat

- White and/or sweetened breakfast cereals (e.g. Frosties, Shreddies, Sugar Puffs, Coco Pops, Alpen muesli)
- Biscuits and breakfast bars (e.g. Jordan's Original Crunchie Bars, Kellogg's Nutrigrain Morning Bars)
- Cream crackers
- Pastries and pies
- White rice (e.g. quick-cook or long-grain but *not* basmati which is low GI)
- Chips or French fries (i.e. potatoes *without* their skins)

Sugars
- Puddings including ice cream
- Chocolate, sweets
- Added sugar in any form! (See 'Recognizing Sugars', overleaf.)

Nicki's Tips

You might not always have your list of 'eats' and 'avoids' with you. A simple rule of thumb is this: 'If it's white, it isn't right!'

If you're having trouble giving up white foods, try eating them with a meal rather than on their own to ensure they don't give your blood-sugar levels a hit. So if I ever want my beloved pick 'n' mix, I try to have some immediately after I've had a good, balanced meal. You still get the enjoyment without the 'spike'.

RECOGNIZING SUGARS

Why: Sugars are hiding everywhere. If something contains sugar it might say it in simple terms on the label, but it might also be in a form you don't recognize.

'Obvious' Sugars

If these were put down in front of you or you saw them on a list of ingredients, you'd probably have a fair idea that they were sugars. These are often referred to as 'overt' sugars:

- Barbados sugar – also called Muscovado – a dark partly refined sugar
- Black treacle – also known as molasses
- Brown sugar
- Burnt sugar – another name for caramel
- Golden syrup
- Honey – a natural combination of glucose, fructose, sucrose and maltose
- Maple syrup
- Raw sugar
- Table sugar – another name for white sugar (sucrose)

'Hidden' Sugars

These sugars – often known as 'covert' sugars – aren't so easy to spot. They often have hard-to-understand chemical names that bear little relation to the word 'sugar':

What to Eat

- Amazake – a purée containing glucose and fructose from fermented rice or millet
- Barley syrup – also known as malt syrup
- Cane juice/sugar/syrup
- Corn syrup/sweetener
- Date sugar
- Dextrose – another name for glucose (also called corn sugar)
- Fructose – naturally occurring fruit sugar. If it's 'intrinsic' (i.e. in the fruit) it's fine, but if it's extrinsic (added to a food later on) then it's still sugar!
- Glucose/glucose syrup
- High-fructose corn syrup
- Demerara
- Disaccharides
- Jaggary – unrefined brown sugar made from palm sap
- Lactose and lactate – milk sugars
- Levulose/lavulose – another name for fructose
- Malt syrup – also known as barley syrup
- Maltose
- Maltodextrin
- Rice sugar

> ### Nicki's Tips
>
> *I bought some organic cola bottles and thought I'd found something sugar-free I could enjoy. But when I looked at the label, I found cane syrup. I looked at my list and discovered this is sugar by another name. It shows you how well hidden these sugars can be. Disappointing – but at least I know!*

SWEETENERS

Some of these are 200 times sweeter than sugar while one, Splenda, is a staggering 600 times sweeter. They are either artificially made or, in the case of sugar alcohols, can be naturally occurring. Splenda is actually made with sucralose, a sweetener made from sugar, but has fewer calories and doesn't affect blood-sugar levels. Artificial 'intense' sweeteners such as aspartame and saccharine are cheap sugar substitutes that are often used in diet and regular soft drinks and low-sugar sweetened products. The good news is that they won't pile on the calories or rot your teeth.

'Bulk' sweeteners such as sorbitol and mannitol are sugar alcohols used, for example, in sugar-free sweets. But unlike intense sweeteners, they do contain calories (though negligible) and can lead to a slight rise in blood-sugar levels, which isn't ideal for those who have

What to Eat

sensitive blood sugar (such as diabetics or those with insulin resistance). They also have a laxative effect if eaten in quantity. So these sweeteners aren't 'innocent' alternatives to sugar, and if you are trying to get your sweet tooth under control, they aren't going to be a great help.

- Acesulfame-K (E950) – an artificial sweetener
- Alitame – an artificial sweetener
- Aspartame (E951) – an artificial sweetener
- Canderel – a trade name for the artificial sweetener aspartame
- Cyclamates (E952) – an artificial sweetener
- Isomalt (E953) – a mixture of sugar 'alcohols', either naturally occurring or manmade
- Lactitol (E966) – a sugar 'alcohol'
- Malitol/malitol syrup (E965) – a sugar 'alcohol'
- Mannitol (Manna sugar) (E421) – a sugar 'alcohol'
- Neotame – an artificial sweetener
- Neohesperidine DC (E959) – an artificial sweetener
- Nutrasweet – a trade name for aspartame
- Saccharin (E954) – an artificial sweetener
- Sorbitol/Sorbitol syrup (E420) – a sugar 'alcohol'
- Splenda – an artificial sweetener made with sucralose
- Sucralose – an artificial sweetener made from sugar
- Sucrose
- Stevia – a herb which can be used as a sweetener
- Thaumatin (E957) – an artificial sweetener

SUGAR ADDICTS' DIET

- Total invert sugar – a liquid sweetener made from sucrose
- Turbinado – a refined 'raw' sugar
- Xylitol (E967) – a sugar 'alcohol'

> ### Nicki's Tips
>
> *It's not always easy to spot sugar. But when you're looking at ingredients, if it's got something ending in '-ose' in it, like glucose or sucrose, you're looking at a sugar. Having problems remembering it? Think of this: 'Too much '-ose' and you won't see your toes!'*

DRINK MORE LIQUIDS

Why: We need water to keep our bodies ticking over. It's needed for metabolism (breaking down food and using it) and for getting rid of toxins. It's also needed in our nervous system for the proper functioning of brain chemicals like serotonin and endorphins, and without it the production of these is impaired. Our bodies are 55–65 per cent water, which is why we need to keep those levels topped up.

We get some of our water from food but we need between 1.5 and 2 litres of additional fluid a day – roughly 8–10 glasses – and an extra half a litre during hot weather or if we exercise. Unfortunately, when we say 'liquids' we don't mean beer, wine, gin or any other alcoholic drink. In theory, tea and coffee count towards your total. Despite what people think, if you don't go over your usual daily total, they won't cause you to lose water. But before you reach for that latte, we've some bad news. We're advising you to try and cut down on tea and coffee because they are stimulants that affect your blood-sugar balancing mechanisms. While they might hydrate, they're not helping to get your sugar cravings under control. **Ideally you should be experimenting with water, herb teas, low-fat milk and watered-down fruit juice (concentrated fruit juice is high GI).**

How to Boost Your Fluid Intake
- **Drink the equivalent of 8–10 glasses of water a day.** Remember, this can be water, fruit/herb teas, low-fat milk, rice milk, soya milk, smoothies or watered-down fruit juice (vegetable juice doesn't need to be watered down). Boosting your fluid intake doesn't have to be boring.
- **Make your water more interesting.** Squirt a drop of lemon juice into it (Jif Lemon is fine) or squeeze in some lime. A few drops of pure vanilla essence can also make for a different taste.
- **Try fruit or herb teas.** Make your own by putting five peppermint leaves into a mug and pouring boiling water on top.
- **Make a fruity thirst-quencher.** Make a herb tea (we

like the London Fruit & Herb Company's Apple Bliss), cool it down and put it in a bottle in the fridge. Add some ice cubes and you've got a great fruity thirst-quencher.
- **Make ice lollies**. Use cooled-down herb teas (the berry varieties such as strawberry and raspberry are especially good). Another option is to use half water, half fruit juice so you get the flavour without the sugar 'spike'.
- **Dilute your fruit juice**. Fruit juice is fine but can cause a rise then dip in blood-sugar levels if drunk concentrated. Mix half and half with water to minimize the effect.
- **Eat more fruit and veg**. Yes, we know you're always being told this. But as well as providing you with vital nutrients such as vitamins, they also consist of 90 per cent water. Food gives us 500–800ml of water per day.
- **Enjoy tea substitutes**. Rooibos (pronounced roy-bosh) tea brews up just like normal tea but is caffeine-free and high in antioxidants to boost the immune system. It doesn't taste exactly like tea but you'll be doing yourself the power of good if you can learn to love it and get those stimulants out of your diet.
- **'Cheating coffee'**. We've really got into Barleycup, a caffeine-free coffee substitute made from roasted barley, rye and chicory. Hint: use two teaspoons rather than the one they tell you to – it'll give you that strong flavour you enjoy so much from coffee.

What to Eat

Nicki's Tips

If you look at a 1.5 litre bottle of water and think, 'I'm going to drink that in a day!', play tricks on yourself by filling six small bottles with water and leaving them around the place to drink instead. Keep one in the car to swig when you're parked up, one in your bag and another by your computer. Before you know it, you'll have drunk the lot! Another way is to buy a desk water dispenser, which contains eight glasses of water (£9.99: www.iwantoneofthose.co.uk)

Another trick that works for me is to have a glass of water every hour, on the hour, from the moment I get to work – so one at 9am and each hour until 4pm.

I know herb teas don't always have a great press, but I've discovered some fantastic ones. Twinings Selection Herbal Infusions come in wonderful flavours including a blackcurrant, ginseng and vanilla variety. It's like a blackcurrant drink – but without the calories.

Cool water-based drinks can be made more interesting if they're carbonated. Either use sparkling mineral water as a base or carbonate using a Sodastream.

- **Have a Virgin Mary**. Tomato juice isn't always a favourite tipple but add Tabasco, horseradish and a bit of celery salt to it and pretend you're having a Bloody

Mary – without the alcohol. A good pre-prepared vegetable drink is V8. Can't stomach it? Put it in a bowl and imagine you're drinking a cool, summer soup. You could even put some chopped cucumber, onion and tomato in it and make it into a Spanish-style gazpacho. You'll soon find yourself loving it.

EAT THE 'RIGHT FATS'

Why: We're all obsessed with eating low-fat foods. The message that 'fats are bad' was started by the American government in the early 1990s to try and get people to have less saturated fat in their diets. Saturated fats are found in red meats and processed meat products such as sausages. The trouble was that the message didn't explain that some fats are, in fact, good.

The good fats in question are essential fatty acids (EFAs) – Omega 3 and Omega 6. Omega 3s are found in greatest quantity in oily fish, while Omega 6s are found most commonly in nuts and seed oils, or the nuts and seeds themselves. Incorporating these fats into your diet is an important part of beating your sugar addiction. Of course, all fats can make you put on weight if eaten in too great a quantity. But you should know that, in the right quantities in your diet, these EFAs may actually help you to slim down and achieve better health.

These EFAs are known to help improve insulin resistance, maintain lean body weight and improve blood-glucose balance. They also help lower cholesterol

What to Eat

and thin the blood, reducing your risk of heart disease. One study found that dieters who ate almonds – rich in Omega 6 fatty acids – every day for six months lost seven per cent more weight and ten per cent more body fat than those who avoided nuts altogether. Not convinced? These fats also give you soft skin, shiny hair and strong nails.

How to Get the Right Fats

- **Get more EFAs in your diet**. As you'll see below, they are in all kinds of foods.
- **Cook with olive oil**. Switch your cooking oil from sunflower, vegetable or lard to olive oil, which is far better for you. Olive oil is a monounsaturated oil, which makes it less prone to heat damage when you cook with it. Heat-damaged oil can increase your risk of a range of conditions such as heart disease.
- **Avoid foods containing 'hydrogenated' fats**. You'll often see 'hydrogenated fat' or 'hydrogenated vegetable oil' on the packaging of biscuits, cakes, pastry, margarine and other processed foods. Hydrogenation is a process that turns oil solid (i.e. into fat) so it can be used to extend shelf life and make solid foods from a liquid, such as margarine. The trouble is this process leads to so-called trans fats which have no nutritional benefits and can, in fact, be harmful. They raise levels of 'bad' blood cholesterol as well as disrupting insulin receptors, which means

your body releases more insulin to compensate. The Food Standards Agency says there's some evidence to suggest that the effects of these trans fats may be worse than saturated fats. Try to limit your intake of foods containing these 'hydrogenated' fats – a good rule of thumb is that if you reduce your intake of sweet processed foods such as cakes and biscuits, you'll also be cutting your intake of hydrogenated and, therefore, trans fats. Look for margarines that don't contain hydrogenated fats, such as the Pure range e.g. Pure with Sunflower Margarine (www.purespreads.com). These taste the same as other margarines and can be used for cooking and baking, including our recipes.

- **Eat fish**. The official recommendation for oily fish is a maximum of two portions a week for women of childbearing age and girls, and up to four portions a week for men, boys and women past childbearing age. If you can't stomach it, consider taking a daily fish oil supplement. Some varieties also contain Omega 6 oils (found in nuts).
- **Eat nuts**. Every day, have a portion (¼–½ a cup) of nuts and/or seeds for your Omega 6 oils. Nuts are going to be an important snack source for you (see Chapter 9).

Where to Find Omega 3 and 6 Oils
- **Omega 3 oils:** These are found in oily fish (e.g.

salmon, sardines, mackerel, fresh tuna and sea bass), in just a handful of plant sources (linseed/flax oil and seeds, and pumpkin seeds) and in small amounts in green leafy veg.
- **Omega 6 oils:** These are found in nuts and seeds, or the oil from nuts and seeds. But before you go cracking open the cashews, you should know that some nuts and seeds have higher levels of these oils than others. Here's a list of the nuts and seeds highest in Omega 6 oils through to the lowest (from *The Insulin Factor* by Antony J Haynes, Thorsons):

SOURCES OF OMEGA 6 OIL

Highest in Omega 6   Sunflower (60 per cent of oil = Omega 6)

Walnut
Pumpkin
Sesame
Peanut
Brazil
Pecan
Almond
Hazelnut
Linseed
Cashew

Lowest in Omega 6   Coconut   (3 per cent of oil = Omega 6)

Omega 6 oils are also found in sunflower, soya, corn/maize and soya oils, as well as evening primrose oil and blackcurrant seed oil.

Nicki's Tips

If you don't like oily fish but want Omega 3 oils, try eating a handful of pumpkin seeds each day to get your quota. They also provide more than enough beneficial Omega 6 oils.

Another great way of getting Omega 3 is through Columbus Eggs. Each egg gives you half your daily recommended intake of Omega 3s (www.columbuseggs.com)

Soya and linseed breads are good sources of Omega 3 and 6 oils. Plus they are grainy breads so a good source of complex carbs (www.burgen.co.uk)

There are lots of different nuts to choose from, so if you don't like the taste of one sort, try another. Almonds have quite a sweet taste so are great if you need a sweet fix, while Brazil nuts are rich-tasting – a good choice if you're in need of a savoury taste.

When it comes to eating oily fish, don't panic – a can of salmon counts. Canned tuna doesn't but it's still a good, easy source of protein.

A great 'find' for me is Cool Oil from The Groovy Food Company. It's a blend of organic seed oils mixed to give you the perfect balance of Omega 3 and 6. All you need is a spoonful each day – you can drizzle it into your cereal, shake it in with salad dressing or even put it in a smoothie. If you do this you can't even taste it (www.groovyfood.co.uk)

If you don't like the taste of olive oil, use half olive and half sunflower oil to begin with (Sainsbury's do a version of this or mix it yourself). When choosing olive oil, the paler the colour the milder the flavour. The dark green one is best for you, as this is 'cold-pressed' and as pure as it can be. But any olive oil is good for you.

9
How to Eat

How you eat is just as important as what you eat. Eating at random times or waiting until you're really hungry are habits that can leave you feeling light-headed and craving sugar to make you feel human again. Eat the right things at the right time and you can learn to be more in control of your food, rather than it controlling you. The list of actions in this chapter will be incorporated into the 21-day plan:

1. Eat regularly
2. Know your portions
3. Eat the right carbs with protein
4. Eat breakfast
5. Pick the right snacks
6. Eat at bedtime

EAT REGULARLY
Why: Eating the right foods regularly is vital if you're going to beat your sugar cravings. It's also essential if you're trying to lose weight, strange as it may seem. If

you eat regularly, your body won't be forced to 'dump' insulin into the bloodstream in large amounts, as it would if you had just a couple of big meals a day. As we explained in Chapter 4, large levels of insulin lead to a corresponding sugar dip and a desire to eat more sugar to feel better again. Eat little and often and you won't feel hungry and inclined to binge on comfort foods like stodgy carbs and sugar.

How to Eat Regularly

- **Plan your food 'slots'.** Make sure you have these food 'slots' planned each day: breakfast, mid-morning snack, lunch, mid-afternoon snack, dinner, bedtime snack. This might sound bizarre but many of us do actually decide to skip meals (especially if we're trying to lose weight) or find we've nowhere to get food because of poor planning.
- **Don't miss a meal.** Try to eat each of these meals and snacks – they're there for a purpose, to ensure your blood-sugar levels don't drop. If you don't feel hungry around the allotted time, at least have a good snack with you to eat when you do (see the snacks section in the next chapter).

> **Nicki's Tips**
>
> *If you know you'll be on the go all day and won't have time for a proper meal, make sure you have a good complex carb and protein snack. This could even be a PJ Mooothie with an apple – the yoghurt in the smoothie provides protein while the apple provides the complex carbs.*

KNOW YOUR PORTIONS

Why: To make sure you're getting the right foods in the right proportions! You often hear people talking about 'portions', whether it's fruit and veg or a protein like meat. But how do you know what a portion is? Research shows that one in three adults believes a tablespoon of strawberry jam is a portion of fruit. And one in ten mothers thinks orange squash contributes to the recommended five fruit and veg a day.

Around 50 food and drink manufacturers and suppliers have been licensed to put a logo on their packaging, telling us how many portions are in the product. But most of the time it's up to us to judge portion sizes (and, besides, these guidelines don't tell you how much of a 'portion' of other ingredients, such as protein, are in there). There are some official portion recommendations such as two portions of fish a week and five-plus portions of fruit and veg a day, but they don't tend to exist for other food groups. We suggest the following daily amounts for good nutrition:

- 2–3 portions of protein foods
- 2–3 portions of low-fat dairy foods
- 5 portions of complex carbs
- 5-plus portions of fruit and veg

You'll see that this corresponds to the lists below but also to the 21-day meal plan in Chapter 13. Each day, the foods add up to between 1,500 and 2,000 calories – perfect for a good steady weight loss in combination with regular exercises such as Nicki's routine (see Chapter 10).

Here are some guidelines on what a 'portion' actually is. Remember, the key is variety because the more food types you have, the better your nutrition will be. So, for example, although you're allowed 2–3 portions of protein foods daily, we're not suggesting you achieve that by eating six eggs … **Always remember, variety is not only the spice of life, it's the key to better nutrition, too!**

Protein (2–3 portions daily)
What is a Portion?

1 small can of tuna or salmon (100g) or half an ordinary can
2 eggs

How to Eat

1 salmon or other fish fillet (about 100g)

2 Quorn sausages

1 medium chicken breast (about 200g)

Around 100g of mince (turkey or Quorn)

2 tbsp of fat-reduced houmous

4 tbsp (120g) of pulses (e.g. red kidney beans)

2 tsp peanut butter

100g tofu

2–3 slices of ham, chicken roll, Quorn meat substitute slices

Low-fat Milk and Dairy (2–3 portions daily)
What is a Portion?

3 tbsp plain yoghurt (just under 100g)

200ml glass of low-fat milk

30g of Edam cheese

2 tbsp low-fat cream cheese (e.g. Philadelphia light)

125g cottage cheese (half a medium-sized pot)

Nicki's Tips

Try to include both animal and vegetable sources of protein in your diet to ensure you get as wide a range of amino acids (the 'building blocks' of proteins that are essential for good health) as possible.

Complex Carbs (around 5 portions daily)
What is a Portion?

- 2 small baked potatoes (100g)
- 1 sweet potato, baked (100g)
- 2 slices of grainy bread
- ½ a cup of brown or basmati rice (75g)
- 75g egg noodles (cooked weight)
- ½ a cup of oats (100g)
- 1 pitta bread (or two small round ones)
- 100g pasta (cooked weight)
- 4 Ryvitas
- Home-made unsweetened popcorn
- ½ cup of green peas (75g)
- 100g sweetcorn
- 40g popcorn

Fruit and Veg (at least 5 portions a day)
What is a Portion?
Note: one portion should be about 80g.

- 1 apple, banana, pear or orange
- 2 small fruits (e.g. plums or satsumas)
- 1 slice of large fruit (e.g. pineapple or melon)
- ½ a grapefruit or avocado
- 3 tbsp of cooked vegetables (raw, cooked, frozen or tinned)
- 1 handful of dried fruit
- 3 heaped tbsp of fruit salad (fresh, stewed or tinned in fruit juice)

How to Eat

Small bowl of salad
1 glass (150ml) of fruit juice (Note: however much you drink, fruit juice counts as a maximum of 1 portion a day)

> ### Nicki's Tips
>
> *Don't forget, potato isn't counted as a portion of fruit and veg – it's a carbohydrate. So, for example, if you have tuna with a jacket potato and salad, the potato doesn't count as your fruit and veg but your complex carb*
>
> *Keep an eye out for sugar when you're buying dairy produce like cottage cheese and yoghurt. I was surprised to find that some contain sugar where you least expect it. I didn't find it in 'sweet' varieties like pineapple cottage cheese but in 'savoury' ones like Sainsbury's chargrilled vegetables cottage cheese, and Be Good To Yourself prawn cocktail cottage cheese and coronation chicken cottage cheese.*
>
> *Watch out when you're choosing sandwich fillings like turkey slices. I found sugar lurking in some of them – Bernard Matthews premium Norfolk turkey breast had lactose (a type of sugar) in it.*

EAT THE RIGHT CARBS WITH PROTEIN

Why: To help regulate blood sugar levels. Remember the blood-sugar roller coaster in Chapter 3? If you eat sugar or 'sneaky' sugar (refined carbohydrates) on their own, you experience a sugar 'high' where you have loads of energy followed shortly by a 'dip' caused by plummeting blood-sugar levels. One of the ways you can counteract this dip is to look at how you eat as well as what you eat.

Eat complex carbohydrates and protein together. They have a different effect on the body than eating them separately. When you eat them together, the protein slows down the rate at which food empties from the stomach into the small intestine. This reduces the rate at which carbohydrates are broken down in the small intestine. In other words, **eating complex carbs and protein together can really help to slow down the rate at which glucose gets into your blood, so you're less susceptible to severe blood-sugar highs and lows.**

How to Eat Complex Carbs with Protein

- **Eat carbs and protein or dairy for breakfast, lunch and dinner.** As we've seen above, each day you need to be eating 2–3 portions of protein, 2–3 portions of dairy, 5 portions of carbohydrates and at least 5 portions of fruit and veg. For each meal – that includes breakfast, lunch and dinner – you should be having one carb portion, at least one fruit or veg portion and one portion of either protein or dairy.

Lunch and Dinner Examples

- Jacket potato with a protein filling – e.g. Quorn sausage casserole (with tomatoes and apple), tuna with sweetcorn and mayonnaise, low-fat cream cheese and baked beans
- Vegetarian lasagne with green salad
- Fresh grilled tuna with sweet potato wedges and salad
- Feta, olive and baby new potato salad
- Turkey mince or Quorn bolognaise with pasta and salad
- Chicken and cashew stir-fry with egg noodles
- Chilli bean wraps
- Turkey, lettuce and tomato sandwich on grainy bread
- Egg roll with yoghurt mayonnaise and cucumber
- Grated Edam, apple and beetroot sandwich

For these and other delicious recipes, see Chapter 15. For breakfast examples, see below.

- **Follow Nicki's meal plan**. In her weekly meal plan in Chapter 13, Nicki goes through three weeks' typical meals. If you're not sure how to combine carbs with protein, take a look at how she's done it.

> ### Nicki's Tips
>
> *I have a 'carb shelf' in my cupboard and a 'protein shelf' in my fridge so I know that if I go to one, I also have to go to the other to balance it out! This goes for meals and snacks. Leave a sticky note saying 'Don't forget carbs' or 'Don't forget protein' in each of these places.*
>
> *Make a list of carbs and proteins to buy at the supermarket and put the lists next to each other. That way, you can look from one to the other and see which foods are likely to combine well for snacks and meals.*

EAT BREAKFAST

Why: To restore blood-sugar levels after night-time and set you up for the day. Eating might be the last thing you feel like doing when you wake up, but it really is the most important meal of the day. You're literally 'breaking the fast', replacing nutrients that have been used up during the night. You need food to replace carbohydrates used by your brain and to kick-start your metabolism which has slowed down during sleep. Not only that, **but research has shown that people who skip the first meal of the day are more likely to snack on unhealthy foods throughout the morning.**

Breakfast Tips

- **Combine carbs and protein or dairy**. Many of us avoid eating protein at breakfast, either because we're weight-watching and convinced it's fattening or because we can't stomach it. But it's as important to get the protein and carb proportions right for breakfast as it is for the other meals of the day. Have one portion of carbs with one portion of protein or dairy plus at least one portion of fruit or veg. For example, two slices of grainy toast, two scrambled eggs with a chopped tomato plus a glass of diluted fresh orange juice. For more breakfast examples, see the 21-day eating plan in Chapter 13.
- **Eat the right cereals**. There are lots of breakfast cereals out that may be 'fortified with vitamins and minerals' but they're also packed full of sugar. One popular cereal brand contains sugar, partially inverted brown sugar syrup, honey and dextrose. That's four different types of sugar, not to mention 'sneaky' sugars like refined cereals and maize starch. Even ones you think should be sugar-free often contain sugar.

Cereals You Can Eat

No added sugar muesli – e.g. Alpen no added sugar, Sainsbury's no added salt or sugar Swiss-style muesli, Sainsbury's wholewheat muesli, Jordan's organic muesli, Jordan's natural muesli, Whole Earth organic Swiss-style muesli

Shredded wheat – e.g. Nestlé Shredded Wheat and Shredded Wheat Bitesize
Instant hot oat cereal – unsweetened versions, e.g. Sainsbury's instant hot oat cereal, Ready Brek
Porridge – e.g. Scots porridge oats, Jordan's organic porridge oats, Conservation Grade porridge oats

Cereals You Should Avoid
Sweetened mueslis – e.g. Alpen Original – plus other mueslis such as Alpen, Jordan's Crunchy Crisp, Sainsbury's Swiss-style muesli
'Diet style' cereals – e.g. Special K, Kellogg's Just Right Rice Krispies
Corn Flakes – plus Honey Nut Corn Flakes
Sweetened shredded wheat – e.g. Nestlé Shredded Wheat Fruitful, Nestlé Shreddies, Sainsbury's Apricot Wheats
'Children's style' cereals – Sugar Puffs, Frosties, Coco Pops, Honey Nut Loops, Cheerios, Golden Nuggets
Sweetened bran cereals – e.g. All Bran, Bran Flakes, Sainsbury's oat and bran flakes
Sweetened instant hot oat cereals – e.g. Quaker Oatso Simple

And any others that list 'sugar' in the ingredients (or sugar by any other name found in the list in Chapter 7).

How to Eat

> **Nicki's Tips**
>
> *If you look at the ingredients of many cereals, it's easy to think you're choosing something sugar-free when you're not. Remember, corn syrup and dextrose are still sugars. Also, if you've found an organic cereal that contains organic sugar, it's still sugar!*

- **Think outside the box**. When it comes to breakfast, think outside the box, including the cereal box. Breakfast doesn't have to be a conventional meal – if you feel like eating one of the snacks or lunch options for breakfast, like cheese and apple, then go for it, even if it's something you'd normally associate with a different time of the day. The important thing is to make sure it's a complex carb and protein combination, and one you can actually face eating! The choices are endless.
- **Go 'liquid' if you can't eat solids**. If breakfast is a real no-no, then choose a liquid version. Try a smoothie but make sure it contains yoghurt as well as fruit as this will give you the carbs and protein you need. See Chapter 15 for smoothie recipes or choose a good-quality commercial product. We like PJ Mooothies (www.p-j.co.uk) or Innocent Thickies (www.innocentdrinks.co.uk) although these contain a dash of honey. If you can handle it, add a teaspoon of

sesame seeds for extra protein or munch your way through six small almonds.

Here is a 'taster' of some of the delicious breakfast ideas you'll find in Chapter 13.

- Toasted grainy bread with peanut butter and a glass of orange juice
- Cinnamon sultana toast
- Banana and almond smoothie
- Granary toast with scrambled egg and smoked salmon
- Pear and peach smoothie
- 'Meaty' omelette, toast and fruit juice
- Quorn sausage sandwich

Nicki's Tips

If you're having real problems at first with the no-sugar cereals, add a little sweetener. At least you are deciding to add the sweetness – when it's down to the manufacturer, you have to eat the sugar you're given. And it's often hard to know exactly how much that is.

Can't stomach breakfast or even a smoothie? Make sure you have one of the carb and protein snack combinations with you to eat by 10am. If you leave it any later than this, you're likely to get a sugar low and will probably end up bingeing.

PICK THE RIGHT SNACKS

Some people say you shouldn't be eating snacks because it might encourage you to graze throughout the day. But if you're feeling hungry in between meals, you're far more likely to give in and go straight to the vending machine. Having good-quality snacks ready throughout the day is not only good for your blood-sugar levels, it also gives you a psychological boost. No one likes to think they're being starved! Remember, a snack isn't a whole meal – it's a 'mini' meal to stop your blood-sugar roller coaster dipping like mad.

Tips for Good Snacking

- **Combine carbs and protein or dairy for snacking**. Again, the principle is to eat carbs and protein (or dairy) together. But as this is a snack, we're not talking about the same size portions as for a meal. The 21-day meal plan in Chapter 13 is well-balanced for protein, carbohydrate, fruit and veg and dairy, but there are still some portions left over each day for your snacks. In other words, if you stick to the right snacks, you won't be going over the allowed amount and the diet will still work (whether you're on it to normalize blood-sugar levels and/or to lose weight).
- **Know your allowances**. Each day you're allowed three snacks – one in between breakfast and lunch, one in the afternoon and one before bed.
- **Get the snack 'balance' right**. After your meals, what

you're left with for your three snacks is *1 portion of dairy*, *1 portion of protein* and *1 portion of carbohydrate*. You're also allowed as much low GI fruit and veg as you like. Look at the lists in 'Know your portions' to remind yourself of the types of foods we're talking about. Remember, these are *in addition* to your meals.
- **How this works**. You can use up your allowances as you like – you'll probably find yourself splitting them up or 'mixing and matching' to make them more interesting and go further. Below we've made lists of snacks, including good shop-bought options. The idea is that you pick one from each list for each of your snacks:

Dairy: 1 per day*

Corn tortilla chips or crudités (e.g. sliced carrot and cucumber, mange tout, baby sweetcorn) with tomato salsa and grated Edam (30g)

Edam cheese (30g) and apple

Half an avocado with 'mayo' and sesame seeds

Home-made smoothie (see recipes plus 'Good Shop-bought Options')

1 slice of cinnamon sultana toast (see recipes)

3 tbsp plain yoghurt and some berries (e.g. strawberries) plus six nuts

2 rye crispbreads plus Cauldron Tangy Soft Cheese and Spinach Pâté (www.cauldronfoods.co.uk, buy from supermarkets and health food shops)

Crispy pepper or celery cheese fillers (see recipes) with 2 tbsp low-fat cheese

PJ Mooothies in strawberry, mango and banana, and peach and vanilla

* Always eat with a carb

How to Eat

Have the following with some plain yoghurt as a good dairy/carb snack:

Granovita Wild Fruit Bar (contains oatflakes)

Granovita Castus Date and Nut Bar

Organix Organic Apricot Fruit and Cereal Bar (www.babyorganix.co.uk)

Protein: 1 per day*

1 slice of grainy toast or 2 oatcakes with peanut butter

2 Ryvitas with Quorn Deli Style ham, turkey or chicken and salad

Handful of nuts (six nuts) and a piece of fruit or sultanas/dried apricots

20g of home-popped popcorn with nuts and dried fruit

1 sliced apple with 2 tsp peanut butter

Crudités and reduced-fat houmous or taramasalata

Sainsbury's Be Good To Yourself mushroom pâté, or tuna pâté (see recipes) with crudités, grainy toast or crisp bread

Half an avocado with mayonnaise (see recipes)

Fruit and Veg: As many low GI fruit and veg per day as you like.

For example:

Canned peaches in juice

Pear

Apple

Plums

Cherries

Dried apricots

* Always eat with a carb

SUGAR ADDICTS' DIET

Mixed berries

Fruit mix (see recipes)

Clearspring Apple and Apricot fruit purée dessert (100 per cent organic fruit purée: www.clearspring.co.uk)

Crudités

Jordan's All Fruit bars (100% fruit)*

La Fruit in blackcurrant, apricot and raspberry – chewy pieces of real fruit

Frutina Real Fruit snack (fruit 'leather' made from real fruit: www.frutina.com)

Nature's Store yoghurt-coated pineapple chunks (from Boots)

- **Remember the 'halfway' rule.** Try to eat your snack about halfway between your regular meals. For example, if you ate breakfast at 7am and you're due to eat lunch at 1pm, have your snack at around 10am. It's not written in stone, but if you're conscious of these timings, you'll be less likely to skip snacks – or splurge on them within minutes of your last meal!
- **Plan ahead with your snacks.** If you know, for example, that your low-sugar time is 3pm, then don't just wait for it to come along. Have a good protein/carb snack ready to eat before the dip takes a grip.

---

* With all these processed fruit products, try not to have them more than once a day. The real thing is always best!

> **Nicki's Tips**
>
> *If you're confused about portion sizes, take one food from each of the lists – dairy, protein and carbs – as well as some fruit and put them on a worktop or table. Work out how you can combine them to make a snack, then divide them into three so you know what your allowance is when each snack time arrives.*
>
> *Don't like peanut butter? Or perhaps you want more variety. There are other nut butters out there to try, including almond butter, cashew butter and hazel butter. Buy them from health-food shops or visit www.meridianfoods.co.uk*

EAT AT BEDTIME

Why: 'Eat at bedtime? They must be *mad!*' we can hear you saying. Well, you've heard correctly. Most people will tell you not to eat before bedtime or you'll have a restless night's sleep as the food lies heavy in your stomach. We're saying you *should* eat before bedtime. We're not talking about a full three-course meal – we mean a snack of the *right* type of food. This will help to ensure you don't get hungry in the night.

Bedtime Snack Suggestions

- **Eat a slow-release carbohydrate food**, in combination, of course, with protein. We recommend some sugar-free muesli, porridge or some potatoes with their skins. This will help to ensure you don't wake in the night, ready to raid the fridge with a rumbling stomach!
- **Get the portion size right**. This isn't a big meal – it's the equivalent to the snacks above so we're talking half a carb portion and half a protein or dairy. For example, a quarter of a cup of porridge, or a slice of grainy bread and a couple of turkey slices.
- **Try turkey**. Turkey is rich in an essential amino acid called tryptophan which helps the body produce vitamin B_6. This in turn helps to produce the sleep-inducing brain chemical, serotonin. Tryptophan works best on an empty stomach, so if you're eating turkey and a complex carb several hours after your evening meal, it's likely to have a better effect than if you ate it, say, as part of a roast dinner. So to aid sleep, make turkey your bedtime protein.

10

Kick Out Sugar with Exercise

WHY EXERCISE?
You may be thinking, 'I'm already changing my diet – why do I need to exercise, too?' **The fact is, fitting exercise or activity into your everyday life has an essential role in healing your sugar addiction.** This is for two main reasons:

1. Exercise evokes a nice slow rise in your beta-endorphins, those wonderful neurotransmitters that boost self-esteem and make you feel optimistic, competent and compassionate – what a great feeling!
2. Exercise makes your body more sensitive to insulin. This helps move the sugar from your blood into your muscles, where it can be used as fuel. When you are overweight, your body does this less efficiently.

This is why activities that produce a slow rise in beta-endorphins will help you feel better and keep feeling better. No rush, no withdrawal symptoms, no cravings.

Activities that have been scientifically documented to raise your beta-endorphin levels slowly include:

- meditation
- yoga
- exercise
- prayer
- up-beat pop music
- making love
- laughing
- listening to Mozart and other classical music

It's our guess that the complete list includes many more activities, even though they haven't been tested in the laboratory or reported in scientific literature. They include dancing, gardening, doing home repairs, walking with your headphones on, bubble baths, candles, even going to the cinema or theatre with a friend. We have named these activities 'BE raisers', or beta-endorphin raisers. Make your own list. You may be surprised at the number of BE raisers you can find.

TWO TYPES OF EXERCISE

There are two types of exercise you should be doing regularly – **cardio** (cardiovascular) training to work your heart, and **resistance** training to develop muscles. Nicki's exercise routine in this chapter is a resistance routine, but before we go into that we'll tell you how to get more cardio training into your life, too.

Cardio Exercise

As well as doing resistance exercises every other day, you should be trying to get an hour's worth of other physical activity each day. This doesn't mean a gruelling hour in the gym, or even an hour's exercise in one go. It means modifying your everyday life to become more active. Here are some examples of how you can do it:

- Walk to the paper shop instead of jumping in the car = 5 minutes
- Get off the bus a stop earlier on the way to and from work = 15 minutes
- Walk the kids to school, or cycle with them = 10 minutes
- Use the stairs instead of jumping in a lift, or walk up the escalator = 5 minutes
- Take the dog for a walk = 30 minutes
  Grand total = 65 minutes of cardio

All these things may sound small and insignificant, but in the fight against flab they can make all the difference in the world. And as you can see from the list above, we're not talking about climbing Everest – just little changes here and there.

Resistance Exercise

This simple and effective exercise routine will help you lose weight and gain confidence. You'll also tone up, add lean muscle definition and improve your posture – essential to helping you look half a stone slimmer instantly!

Your aim is to get maximum results in the minimum time. Even if you already exercise regularly, you'll have reached a plateau if you've been doing the same routine for more than six weeks. The following moves have been Nicki's favourites for years. They work all your major muscle groups and give you a top-to-toe tone-up. They also raise your heart rate (which will get you burning calories), as well as building lean muscle tissue (which won't bulk you up – body builders use specific techniques to achieve that look). Pound for pound, muscle takes up less room than fat, which is why so many women who take up weight-training find they lose weight without even trying. Muscle also uses up more calories than fat for daily maintenance, so the more muscle you have, the more calories you'll burn every day.

In this routine we'll be working the following areas with resistance exercises:

- Chest and upper back
- Shoulders and arms
- Lower body
- Mid-section

Kick Out Sugar with Exercise

Before You Start
All the exercises can be done at home or in a gym. Before you start the routine, make sure you read the following:

- **Find a pair of hand weights**. These should weigh between 1.5kg and 5kg, and they should provide some resistance without feeling like you're straining yourself. You don't have to buy expensive weights – cans of soup, ½ litre plastic bottles filled with water, sandbags or a couple of bricks will do. For some of the exercises you can use luggage. The only criterion is that the weights are comfortable for you to lift repetitively.
- **Warm up**. Start with a five-minute warm-up of power walking or moderate jogging followed by some light stretches. This will help improve your focus and reduce your risk of injury.
- **Stretching out**. Always end a workout by stretching out the areas you've worked, otherwise your muscles will stiffen. It prevents injury and soreness, vital if you're going to make exercise your new routine and not be put off at the first hurdle!

Exercise Tips
- **Do these exercises every other day.** Your body needs time to recover from exercise.

- **Do them in order.** You may be tempted to start your routine with some exercises you like the look of. Stop! Nicki has devised this regime in this order for a purpose, and we're advising you to stick with it. It's vital that you work the muscle groups in the order given – chest and upper back, shoulders and arms, lower body, then mid-section. If you don't do this you'll risk injuring yourself.
- **Do as much or as little as you want.** Ideally you should be doing 20 minutes of these exercises every other day, but if you can only grab five minutes, do it!
- **If you've got five minutes ...** Pick any one exercise from each of the groups (in other words, four exercises). One set of each of these should take you five minutes. So, for example, do one set of: towel fly, chair dip, wall squat and bicycle.
- **If you've got 10 minutes ...** Pick any one exercise from each of the groups (four exercises) and do *two* sets of each of these *or* pick any two exercises from each group and do *one* set.
- **If you've got 20 minutes ...** Pick any one exercise from each of the groups (four exercises) and do *four* sets of each of these *or* pick any four exercises from each group and do *one* set.

Nicki's Tip

As long as you do these exercises in the group order I recommend – chest and upper back, shoulders and arms, lower body, then mid-section – you can do them how you like. You can mix and match them, picking one from the top of the lower-body list and another from the bottom. That way it'll be more interesting ... and you're more likely to stick to it!

Chest and Upper Back

Beginners should do two sets of 10 to 15 reps (repetitions) of each of these exercises. Intermediate and advanced lifters should do three sets, with 8 to 10 reps of each.

STACKED FEET PRESS-UP

a) Kneel on floor, putting one foot on top of the other so only the lower one supports your body. Place hands about shoulder-width apart, palms flat on the floor. Straighten your arms without locking your elbows.

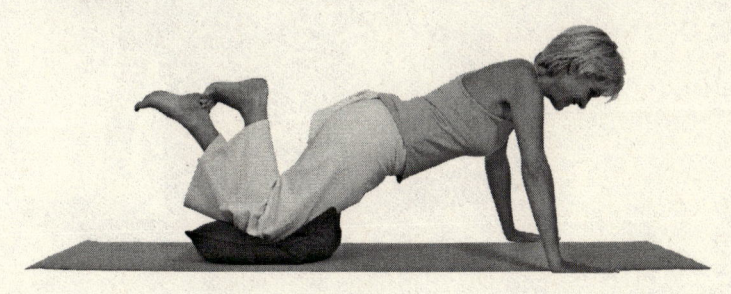

SUGAR ADDICTS' DIET

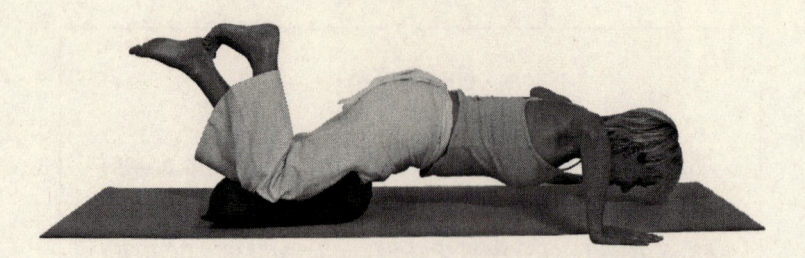

b) Lower your torso until your chest is just a fraction of an inch off the floor. Push yourself back to the starting position.

Variations
- *Slow press-up: Lower your body in an exaggerated slow movement to keep your chest and arm muscles under tension longer.*
- *Stop-and-go press-up: From the top position, go down one-third of the way and stop for 2 or 3 seconds. Lower yourself another third and stop again. When you reach the bottom position, stop a third time before pressing back up quickly.*

TOWEL FLY

a) Assume the press-up position on a hard wood or tiled floor – a rug or mat won't work for this one. Place a small, thick towel under each hand.

Kick Out Sugar with Exercise

b) Keeping a slight bend in your elbows, move your arms up and out to your sides on top of the sliding towels so your hands are in line with your ears. Then use your chest to move the towels back in.

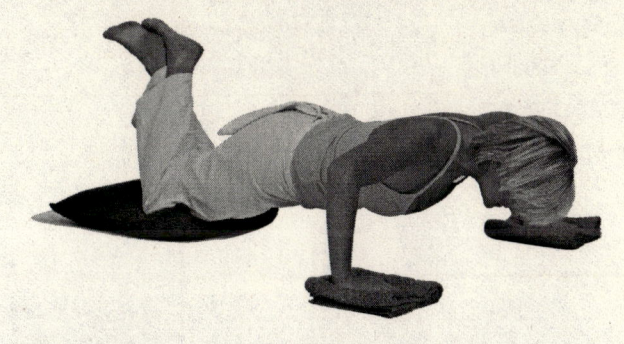

ONE ARM ROW, ELBOW IN

a) Grab a full plastic water or detergent bottle with your non-dominant hand. Place your other hand and knee on a sturdy bench or stool. Plant your other foot flat on the floor and let your working arm hang down slightly ahead of your shoulder, with your palm facing the chair. Keep your back straight.

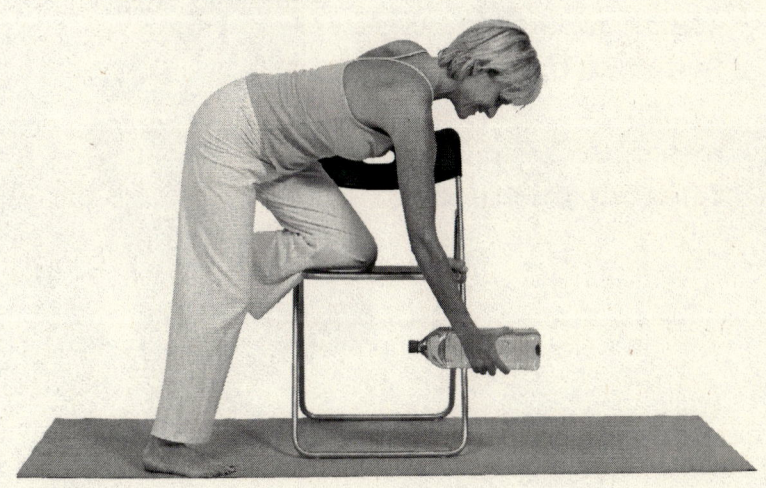

SUGAR ADDICTS' DIET

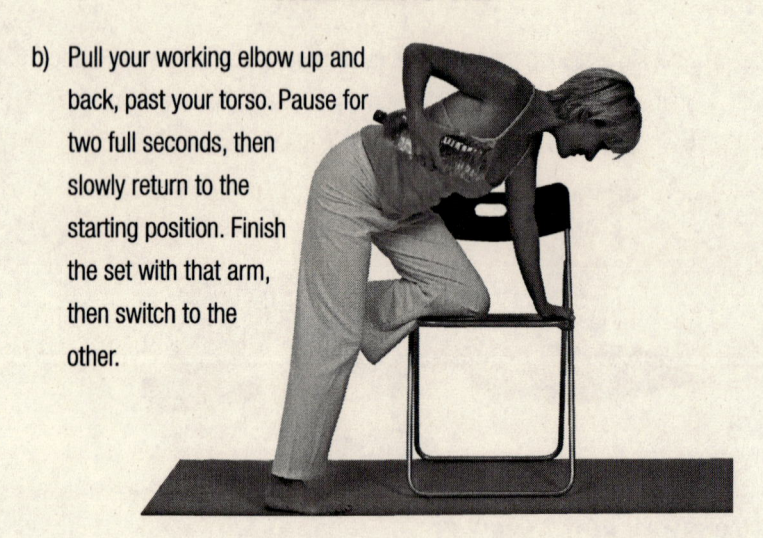

b) Pull your working elbow up and back, past your torso. Pause for two full seconds, then slowly return to the starting position. Finish the set with that arm, then switch to the other.

BENT-OVER ROW

a) Lay a full travel bag in front of you. You can use anything for a weight – luggage, a sandbag, a couple of bricks, whatever. Stand with your legs comfortably apart, then bend over at your hips with your knees bent and your back flat and grab the handles or sides of the weight.

Kick Out Sugar with Exercise

b) Use your back and biceps (front of arm) to pull the weight up to your chest, keeping it close to your body. Pause, then slowly return to the starting position.

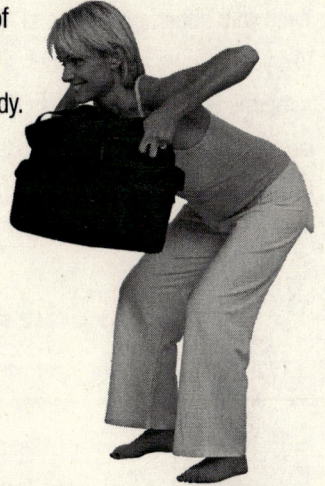

Shoulders and Arms

Beginners should do one or two sets of 10 to 15 reps (repetitions). Those at intermediate and advanced levels can do two or three sets of 8 to 10 reps.

EXTERNAL ROTATION

a) With a small plastic bottle of water or soup tin in each hand, hold your arms out to your sides with your elbows bent at 90 degrees so your upper arms are just a couple of inches below your shoulders and almost parallel to the floor, and your forearms are pointed in towards your torso.

SUGAR ADDICTS' DIET

b) Keep your upper arms still and use your elbows to rotate your forearms up until they are as close to perpendicular to the floor as possible. Return to the starting position.

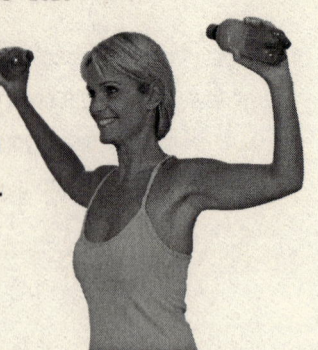

UPRIGHT ROW

a) Fill a gym or travel bag with books or something else heavy enough to create a challenging weight. Hold the bag by its straps with both hands. Let your arms hang straight down, with your hands 30–60cm (12–24in) apart. (The further you place them apart, the easier and more natural the exercise is for your shoulders.)

b) Lift the bag straight up along your torso until your upper arms are parallel to the floor. Pause to feel the contraction in your shoulders and back of your neck, then slowly return to the starting position, staying in control.

Kick Out Sugar with Exercise

CHAIR DIP

a) Hold on to the seat of a sturdy chair behind you, with your knees bent and your feet flat on the floor – as if you were seated in another, invisible chair.

b) Keep your back arched and close to the chair as you slowly lower your body until your upper arms are parallel to the floor. Your torso should remain straight. Pause, then press back up to the starting position.

ONE-ARM TRICEPS EXTENSION

a) Lie on your side with your legs, hips and shoulders stacked over each other. Reach your bottom arm across your body and grab your opposite shoulder. Place your free hand on the floor, in front of your chest.

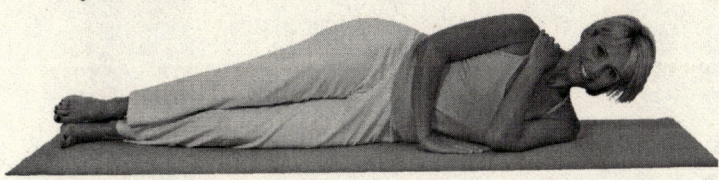

SUGAR ADDICTS' DIET

b) Use your upper triceps to push your entire upper torso off the floor so that only your hips and legs remain in contact with the floor. Return to the starting position. Finish the set with that arm, then switch sides.

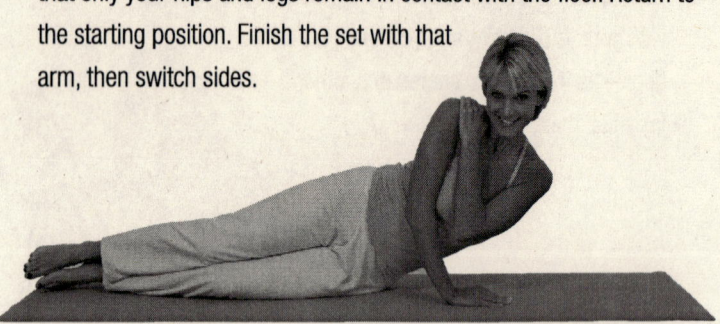

SELF-RESISTANT BICEPS CURLS

a) Stand with your knees slightly bent and your abdomen tucked in, your non-dominant arm down at your side with your palm facing forwards. Put your opposite palm over your wrist.

b) Make a fist with your working hand and execute a biceps curl with that arm whilst resisting it with the other. Shift the resistance on the way so your palm pushes the working arm down. Return to the starting position. Finish your set, then repeat with the other arm doing the work.

Kick Out Sugar with Exercise

TOWEL CURL

a) Fold a large bath towel lengthways a few times and hold it at either end, your palms facing each other, as you stand with your back against a wall. Move your feet out about 30cm (12in) in front of you, and place one of them in the middle of the towel (at the bottom of the U the towel makes as you hold it). Start with both knees slightly bent.

b) With your arms straight down, curl your fists up towards your shoulders while using your foot to resist the movement. Keep your upper arms still and against your body so all the pulling power comes from your elbow joints. Pause at the top, using your arms to resist your leg's attempt to push the towel back down to the floor. Return to the starting position.

Lower Body

Beginners should do one or two sets of 12 to 15 reps (repetitions) of each exercise. Advanced and intermediate lifters should do two to three sets of 12 to 15 reps.

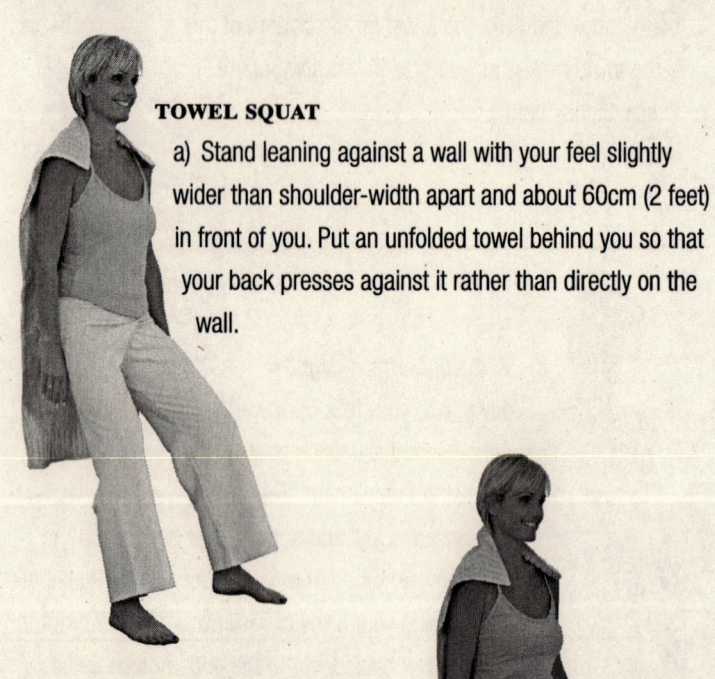

TOWEL SQUAT

a) Stand leaning against a wall with your feet slightly wider than shoulder-width apart and about 60cm (2 feet) in front of you. Put an unfolded towel behind you so that your back presses against it rather than directly on the wall.

b) Bend your knees and let your back slide down the wall along with the towel until your upper thighs are parallel to the floor. Pause, then push yourself back up.

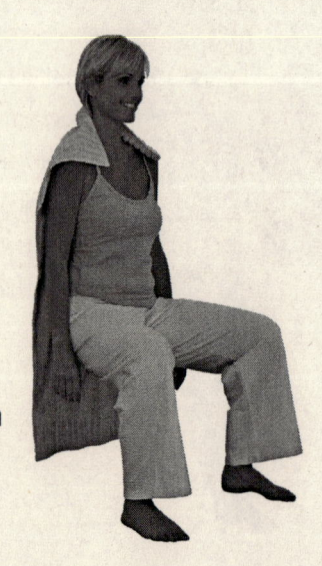

Kick Out Sugar with Exercise

WALL SQUAT

a) Lean back against a wall with your feet 60cm (2 feet) in front of you as in the towel squat – but without the towel.

b) Bend your knees to descend 5–8cm (2–3 in), and freeze there for 30 seconds. Slide down another few inches and stop again for another 30 seconds. Stop two or three more times as you work your way down until your bottom is almost touching the floor. That's the end of the first set.

Variation
- *10-second-stop ski squat: Same exercise, with 10-second stops.*

SUGAR ADDICTS' DIET

LUNGE

a) Stand with both feet together and your hands on your hips.

b) Take a long step forwards so your front foot lands 60cm to 1m (2 to 3 feet) in front of you, and lower your body until the top of your front thigh is parallel to the floor. Your forward knee should be over your toes, not past them. Quickly and forcefully, push yourself back to the starting position.

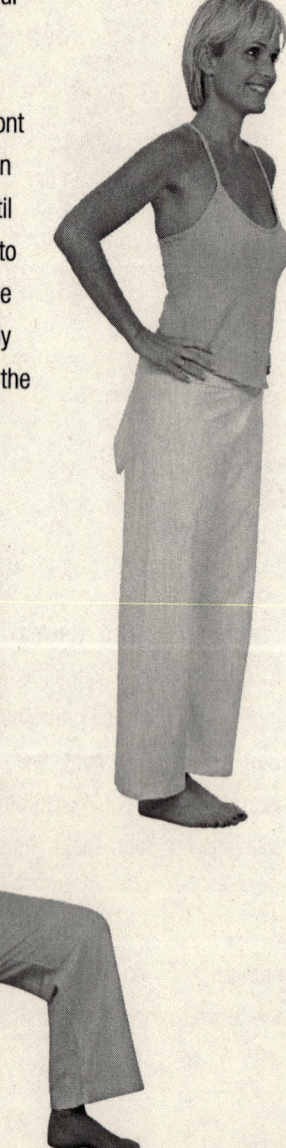

Kick Out Sugar with Exercise

LYING HIP AND THIGH EXTENSION

a) Lie on the floor with your arms at your sides and both heels up on a chair or bench, with your knees bent.

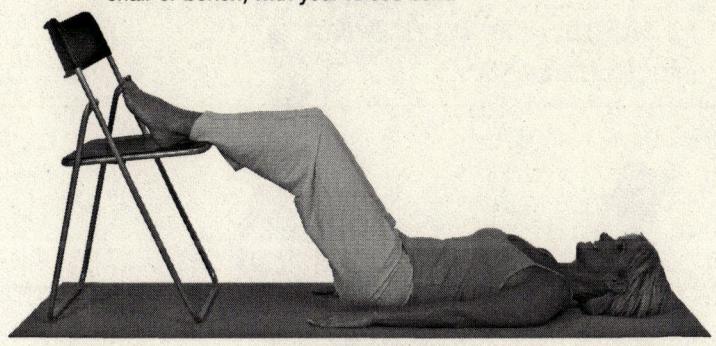

b) Pushing with your buttock muscles and hamstrings, dig your heels down into the seat of the chair and lift your hips until your body forms a ramp that descends from your knees to your shoulders. Pause, then return to the starting position.

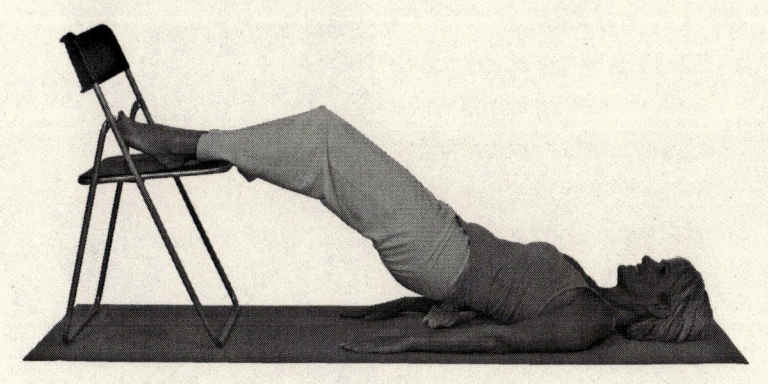

SUGAR ADDICTS' DIET

Variation
- *Elevated-leg lying hip extension: For a greater challenge, straighten one leg and hold it directly over its hip before you lift up. The elevated leg should stay perpendicular to the floor throughout the exercise.*

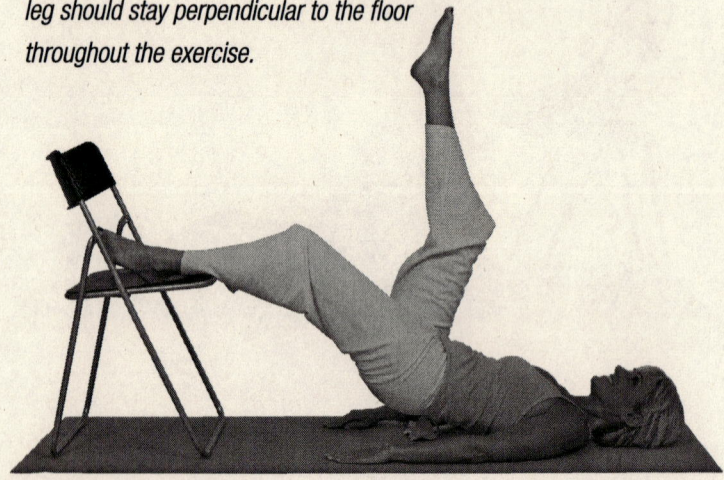

ONE-LEG CALF RAISE

a) Stand with the ball of your non-dominant (weaker) foot on the edge of a step or wooden block 5–8cm (2–3 in) high. Hook your other foot around the back of your non-dominant heel. Hold on to a banister or something sturdy to stay balanced.

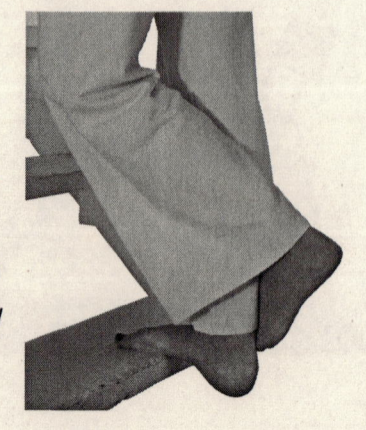

b) Let your non-dominant heel drop as low as it'll go off the step. Then change direction and push off the ball of that foot until the heel is 5–8cm (2–3 in) above the step.

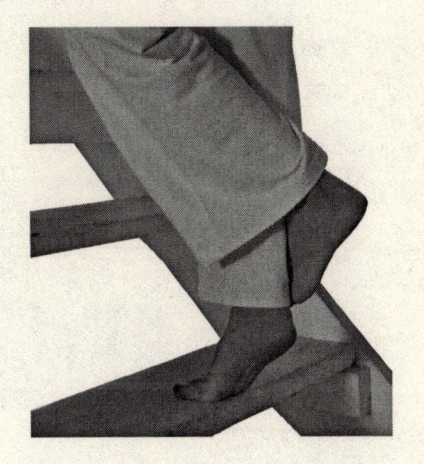

Mid-Section

If you're a beginner, do one set of 10–15 reps (repetitions) per exercise – except for The Vacuum (page 188), when you should do 6–10 reps. If you're more experienced, do two or three sets of 8–10 reps of each chosen exercise.

REVERSE CRUNCH

a) Lie with your arms at your sides. Hold your legs off the floor with your knees bent at a 90-degree angle so your thighs point straight up and your lower legs point straight ahead, parallel to the floor.

SUGAR ADDICTS' DIET

b) Crunch your pelvis towards your rib cage. Your tailbone should rise 5–8cm (2–3 in) off the floor as your knees move towards your chin. Pause, then slowly return to the starting position.

RUSSIAN TWIST

a) Sit with your torso at a 45- to 60-degree angle to the floor (as if you're halfway through a sit-up) and your arms raised directly out in front of you. Bend your knees and keep your feet free, not anchored by anything.

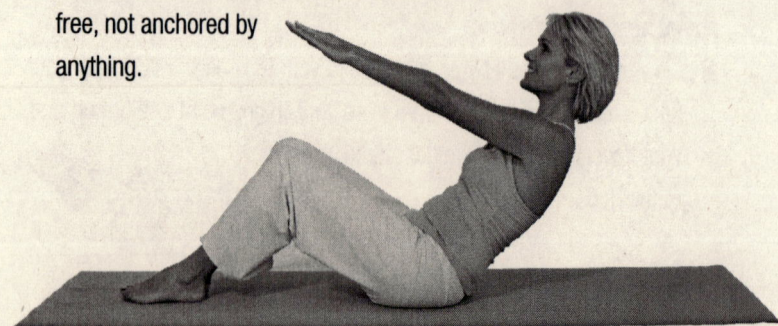

Kick Out Sugar with Exercise

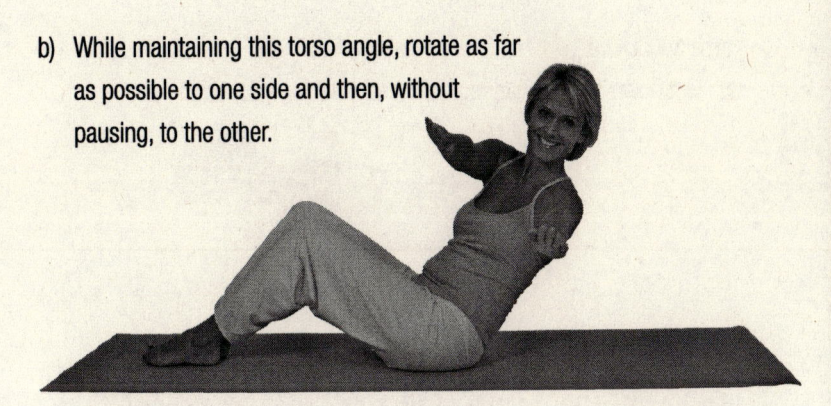

b) While maintaining this torso angle, rotate as far as possible to one side and then, without pausing, to the other.

THE BICYCLE

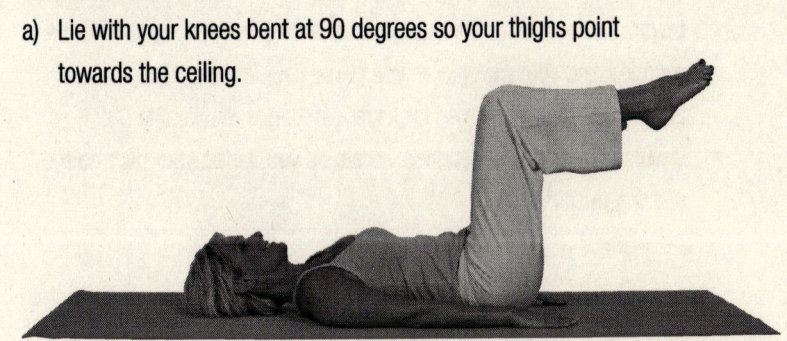

a) Lie with your knees bent at 90 degrees so your thighs point towards the ceiling.

b) Hold your hand behind your ears. Pump your legs back and forth, bicycle-style, as you simultaneously rotate your torso from side to side by moving an armpit (not elbow) up towards the opposite knee.

SUGAR ADDICTS' DIET

THE VACUUM

a) Get down on your hands and knees, keeping your back flat.

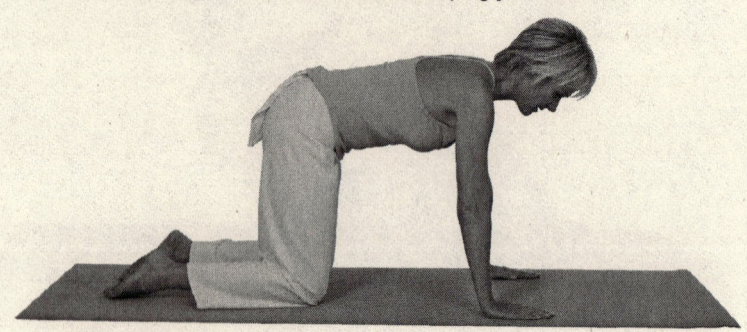

b) Take a deep breath, allowing your stomach to bulge out. Then forcibly exhale and round your back like an angry cat as you lift your navel up towards your spine. When you can exhale no more, keep your back rounded and your navel in as you purse your lips and take shallow breaths through your nose for several seconds. That's one rep; it should take 20 to 30 seconds. Inhale as you flatten your back to the starting position.

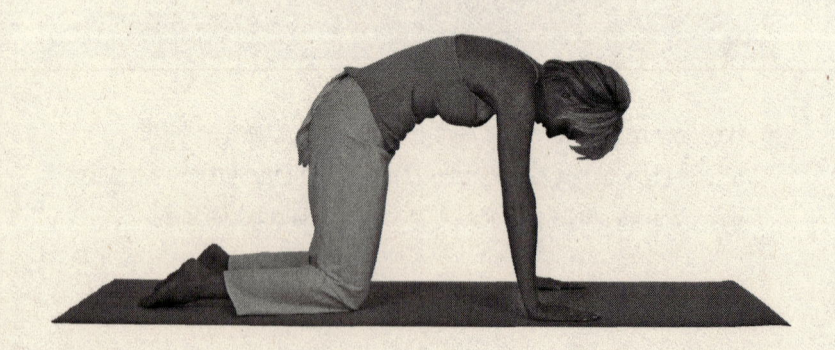

Kick Out Sugar with Exercise

BIRD-DOG

a) Start on all fours, with your knees and toes on the floor and your palms face down in front of you.

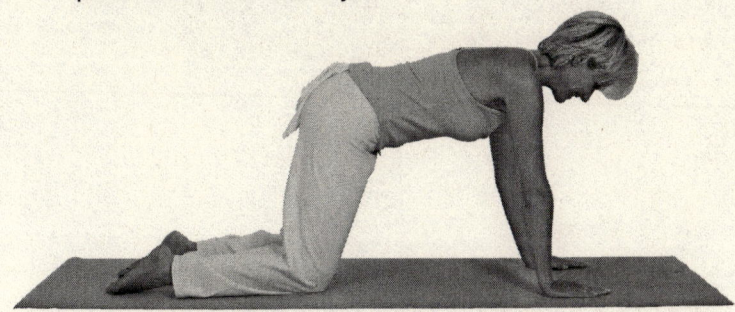

b) Pull in your abdomen, then straighten one arm and the opposite leg, extending both limbs parallel to the floor while keeping your torso and hips in a straight line. Hold for 1 to 5 seconds, then lower your working limbs and repeat with the opposite arm and leg. That's one rep.

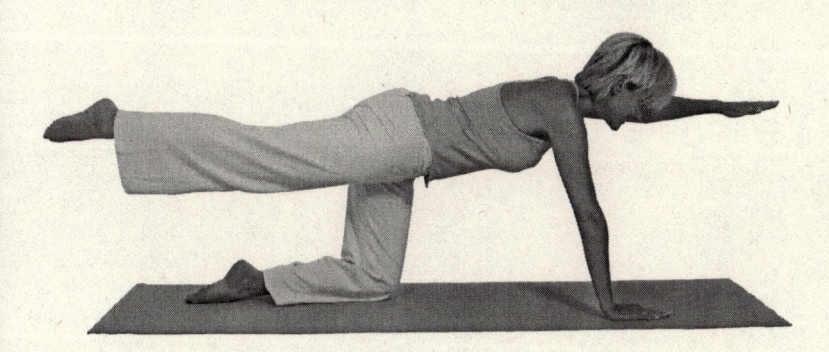

11
Hints and Tips for Giving Up

These are Nicki's hints and tips – things she found useful in her bid to get those extra sugars out of her diet.

HOW TO GET THAT SWEET TASTE
- **Puréed fruit**. You might associate it with baby food, but it really can help you get your sweet 'buzz'. And a little goes a long way – mix a spoonful of puréed pear in with your freshly popped popcorn and cook together for an extra 30 seconds in the microwave for a good semi-sweet snack. We also like Clearspring 100% Fresh Fruit Purées in apple, blueberry, plum and apricot (www.goodnessdirect.co.uk)
- **Buy sugar-free baby food**. We're not saying eat loads of jars of baby food, but if you want a sweet treat – especially if you're 'on the go' – a jar of sugar-free fruit purée can be just what you need. These can also be used like the puréed fruit (above) as a snack with popcorn or plain yoghurt. Watch that they don't contain added sugars such as fructose, sucrose, glucose syrup or honey.

- **Make your own jelly**. Shop-bought sugar-free jellies contain artificial sweeteners, so by eating them you're not reducing your desire for sweet foods. By mixing gelatine or agar-agar (buy it from the supermarket or health-food shop) with a can of fruit in its juice (or just fruit juice if you don't like 'lumpy' jelly) you can make your own sugar-free jelly. Some fruits work better than others – for example, enzymes in fresh pineapple stop jelly from setting. Strawberries and raspberries work well, as do mandarins, pears and peaches.
- **Use cocoa powder**. If you're missing the taste of chocolate, use pure cocoa powder instead. It's not sweet but you'll learn to love its chocolatey taste. Carob powder (buy from supermarkets or health-food shops) is also a good chocolate-tasting option, but check the label for added sugar.
- **Discover flavourings**. Vanilla essence and cinnamon are two of our favourites for helping to give bland foods crying out for sugar that little something 'extra.' For example, use them in porridge or, again, in your popcorn.
- **Make ice cream**. We really mean it! See the recipes section for how to do it using yoghurt or tofu. It's absolutely delicious.
- **Have sweet vegetables**. Carrots, sweetcorn, parsnips and sweet potatoes are all sweet, and they're all foods you can eat (in combination with other foods; see

Hints and Tips for Giving Up

Chapter 8). As a result, they're often used in desserts. Learn to enjoy their sweetness.

GOOD SHOP-BOUGHT OPTIONS
This isn't a list of everything available but it should give you some useful pointers in case you're wondering what you can eat. Chapter 7 tells you how to spot sugars on labels so you can judge for yourself whether a food is on the 'eat' or 'don't eat' list.

Snacks
Jordan's All Fruit bars – 100% fruit (apple and passion fruit and apple and strawberry)
Granovita Wild Fruit bar or snack bar (from Sainsbury's)
Lyme Regis Zap bars (orange and apricot) and Grizzly bars (apricot & honey, banana & sultana, pineapple & papaya and blackcurrant & apple) – from Sainsbury's, Tesco, Waitrose, Boots, Holland and Barrett (www.lymeregisfoods.com)
La Fruit in blackcurrant, apricot and raspberry – chewy pieces of real fruit. A good chewy sweet substitute (visit www.lymeregisfoods.com for range and stockists)
Nature's Store yoghurt-coated pineapple chunks (from Boots)
Sainsbury's Be Good To Yourself mushroom pâté
Cauldron Tangy Soft Cheese and Spinach pâté (try other options from the Cauldron range:

www.cauldronfoods.co.uk), from supermarkets and health-food shops

PJ Mooothies in strawberry, mango and banana, peach and vanilla (organic low-fat bio yoghurt with fruit and juices)

Food Doctor range (www.thefooddoctor.com), available at Tesco

Breakfasts

Sainsbury's no added salt or sugar Swiss-style muesli
Sainsbury's wholewheat muesli
Sainsbury's instant hot oat cereal
Ready Brek
Scots porridge oats
Jordan's organic porridge oats or conservation grade porridge oats

Lunches and Dinners

Heinz curried beans
Old El Paso refried beans
Cauldron spicy Middle Eastern falafel
Quorn sausages
Linda McCartney flame-grilled beefless burgers
Quorn premium burgers with a chargrill seasoning
Quorn peppered steaks
Quorn deli-style turkey, ham and chicken – like sliced meat but low-fat and rich in plant proteins. Delicious!

Hints and Tips for Giving Up

> **Nicki's Tips**
>
> *If you can't stomach really wholesome brown breads, ease your way with a loaf such as Hovis Best of Both, which is soft white bread with added wheatgerm. This will get you used to the concept of brown bread so you can eventually make the change.*
>
> *As well as the usual vegetables, lots of the foods listed above come in frozen form, such as Quorn sausages or chunks, and bags of chicken breasts. I find having these in the freezer makes me more likely to make good food choices because I've got no excuses for not having any in stock! Take your time to look through the freezer department of your supermarket – I guarantee you'll find some useful foods you've previously overlooked.*

USEFUL FLAVOURINGS

- **Cinnamon**. This is a brilliant and entirely sugar-free flavouring. You can buy it either in ground form or as cinnamon sticks which you can infuse to release the flavour. Add it to popcorn, porridge or muesli for extra flavour. Cinnamon doesn't only taste good – studies suggest it enhances the ability of insulin to metabolize glucose, helping to control blood-sugar levels.

- **Vanilla**. If the mention of vanilla makes you think of ice cream and Victoria sponges, take heart – you can still have vanilla without the sugar and fat. In fact, you can use it to flavour our own ice-cream recipe (page 326), or even add it to coffee substitutes for a drink to rival those from high-street coffee shops. But beware – many vanilla flavourings have sugar added to them. Go instead for pure vanilla extract or vanilla pods, which tend to be sugar-free. Check the label before you buy.
- **Mint**. It may be that the only way you're used to having mint is in mint chocolate or with roast lamb. But as well as being a good stomach settler (for example, if you have indigestion), mint is also a great way to flavour foods. Put a mint leaf plus a couple of drops of lemon juice in each compartment of an ice-cube tray and freeze for flavoured ice cubes to make water more interesting. It's also great chopped in fruit salad.
- **Ginger**. This is a great spice for both savoury and sweet dishes (as well as being a traditional remedy for nausea such as morning sickness). Add dried ginger to porridge or oat biscuits (think gingerbread men or ginger cake) for a warming, aromatic taste.

Hints and Tips for Giving Up

KITCHEN GADGETS

- **Popcorn popper** – we like the Rival PP25 popcorn maker, which is a really reasonable £19.99. All it needs is a bit of butter but we've tried it with some olive oil and it works just as well.
- **Blender** – whether it's one of the hand-held ones or a free-standing jug blender, these are great for smoothies and purées. We like the Braun Multiquick range, especially the 3 in 1 (such as the MR4050 HC 3 in 1 blender), which also has attachments so you can chop nuts and seeds, as well as herbs, onions and garlic (so you don't have the smell of it on you all day!). If you have a blender like this, you won't need to bother with separate equipment like a smoothie maker or a juicer, unless you really want to.
- **Coffee grinder**. No doubt you're saying, 'Why would I need one of these if I'm trying to cut down on coffee?' Coffee grinders such as the compact Braun AromaGourmet allow you to chop up nuts and seeds ready to put in foods such as yoghurt. Some people like to have them as well as a blender but if you've got attachments for chopping, you might feel you can do without one of these.
- **Sodastream**. Carbonating your drinks can make them more interesting. Use carbonated (fizzy) water to liven things up, or if you have a Sodastream, use this to add fizz to otherwise still drinks, such as cooled fruit teas.

- **Health grill**. A different way to cook chicken, vegetables or veggie burgers. You can also do toasted sandwiches in it without having to coat the outside in fatty spreads. If you want to use a sandwich toaster, use a pastry brush to brush the bread with olive oil to stop it sticking. Or buy a refillable oil sprayer so you can finely mist extra virgin olive oil onto your food and cookware.
- **Bread maker**. While most diets are probably telling you to cut out bread, you'll soon see this isn't one of them. The right kind of bread made with the right kind of flour and other ingredients can be a good thing. We've started making our own bread and we found it surprisingly easy – just chuck everything in, leave it to cook for a few hours and there it is. And unlike shop-bought breads, you can tell exactly what's gone into them! Yeast needs a bit of sugar to grow – we use a dab of Manuka honey in our bread so at least it has some other nutritional benefits to it.
- **Ice-cream maker**. You can be so inventive with these, freezing yoghurt or even tofu mixtures (sounds horrible, tastes lovely) to produce sugar-free puds. If you don't want to buy one, make sure you have a good sturdy freezable box with a lid (the sort normal ice cream comes in – but don't buy one especially to empty it!) and you can still make frozen desserts.
- **Ice cube makers**. Use ice cube trays or buy a roll of ice cube-maker bags. Fill with fruit juice or cooled

Hints and Tips for Giving Up

fruit tea to make ice lolly 'suckers' or to put in water to make it more interesting.
- **Plastic boxes**. This probably sounds obvious, and no doubt every mum around the country is saying, 'They've *got* to be joking.' But not everyone knows that having plastic containers (such as those you buy at any supermarket or Woolworths) are vital for helping you ensure you always have your snacks or meals to hand. How many times have you gone to the vending machine, canteen or newsagent because you didn't have snacks with you? Well, plastic boxes will help you make sure this doesn't happen again. They come in all kinds of sizes, including tiny ones for those essential nuts and seeds we'll be telling you about (see Lakeland www.lakelandlimited.com for a good range).

Nicki's Tips

You can buy fantastic frozen fruit treat makers. These allow you to skewer cut pieces of fruit and place them in a special container to freeze them. A perfect sugar-free frozen solution for those hot days when only a lolly will seem to do! But if you haven't got one of these to hand, make a brilliant healthy 'lolly' by putting a banana in the freezer for a couple of hours. Take it out, unpeel it and enjoy a refreshing, healthy snack.

When you're making bread, 'supercharge' it and make it extra healthy with a few simple changes. Use olive oil instead of butter, Manuka honey instead of sugar (it's for the yeast!) and Lo Salt instead of the usual table salt. Also, add linseeds and other seeds such as sesame and pumpkin to it and you'll help to boost your daily intake of essential Omega 3 and 6 oils.

12

Coping with Sugar 'Dealers'

You now have the mechanisms to deal with your addiction. As with all addiction, however, temptation will always be around, often when you least expect it. And as with other addictions, the last thing you need is a sugar 'dealer' trying to get you off the straight and narrow. Unfortunately they're everywhere: the friends who say, 'Go on, have a biscuit', the cinemas which entice you to eat ice cream and bags of sweets, the supermarkets with their special offers, and fast food containing 'hidden' sugar.

In all these situations, you could decide to say 'Who cares – it's a special occasion and I'm going to enjoy myself.' Who are we to say you shouldn't let your hair down? But as is so often the case, one piece of cake often turns into two, followed by a sausage roll and a serving of trifle, and before you know it that one treat has become a forbidden feast!

In this chapter we give you mechanisms for coping with these 'dealers' so that you can go to parties, fast-food joints or entertainment venues without feeling like you're waiting to trip up. It's about giving you the power

– through making the right choices and having the tools to say 'no' – to get sugar back on your terms. If you're more in control of your eating habits, you should soon be able to go out and be really happy with that one piece of cake. Use these tips on coping with sugar 'dealers' – whether they're situations, people or places – and you're on your way there.

TEN COMMON SUGAR 'DEALERS'
1. Good Times, Bad Times
The 'Dealers'
- **The 'what the hell' factor.** Special occasions don't come round very often so you may well say, 'Oh what the hell! I'm going to eat what I want.' That would be fine if we had one day of enjoyment and stopped it there. But generally we don't. We see Christmas as several weeks of indulgence, we have Easter eggs hanging round for at least a week and we spend our lives in a constant state of stress so eat sugary foods regularly to make ourselves feel better.
- **The need for a lift.** Whether you're tired and stressed from work, feeling miserable because of relationship problems or upset because of a sad event such as a bereavement, there are those low times in life when sugar seems like your best and only friend. If you're used to eating sugar when you're low, you'll be more tempted than usual to reach for something sweet when sadness or pressure strike.

How to Cope
CHRISTMAS, EASTER AND OTHER BIG HOLIDAYS

- **Stick with the diet's main principles**. Although holidays often mean lots of tempting, sweet foods in the house, the positive side is that you're also likely to have proper, balanced meals with protein and veg. Remember the principle of eating carbohydrates with protein and stick to it. A Christmas dinner or Sunday roast fits in well with this (though avoid the cranberry or mint sauce, unless it's homemade without added sugar).
- **'Buffer' your vices**. We know that once in a while you're going to want something you ideally shouldn't, like something sweet. We've talked to you about using protein and carb meal combinations to help level out blood-sugar. You can also use this to help minimize the effect of stimulants or sugars on your blood-sugar. We're not saying use this all the time or ditch the book and use this device instead. But it *can* be a useful tool for those moments when you can't avoid eating or drinking those treats. If you have to have sweet foods such as chocolate, eat them *with* your meals, rather than on their own as a sneaky snack. Eating them on a full stomach will help reduce the likelihood of them causing a sugar 'high'.
- **Make the most of healthy seasonal foods**. Although different holidays bring with them lots of dubious, sugary foods (such as Christmas cake, mince pies and

Easter chocolate), there are also plenty of good, non-sugary foods associated with those times. For example, Christmas means lots of delicious satsumas and nuts, while a summer barbecue can include lovely fresh fruit salads using special, exotic fruits such as mango and star fruit. At Easter, make one of our sugar-free desserts such as cheesecake so you can eat that while others may be going for the sugared version.

- **Focus on other activities**. These family get-togethers don't have to be all about eating, even though they very often end up as face-stuffing food fests. Put a different focus on the time you have, and when you'd automatically crack open a box of biscuits, crack open a board game instead. Whether it's Monopoly, Who Wants To Be a Millionaire? or even Snakes and Ladders, you'll find you're concentrating so hard that eating (which often comes out of boredom) will be the last thing on your minds.
- **Keep healthy snacks to hand**. If you're tempted but there's no healthy snack to hand, it'll be no surprise if you go for that portion of trifle instead. If you're at home, keep your snack cupboard well stocked, and if you're away, make sure you have something healthy in your handbag or in the car. Faced with temptation, it may be hard to resist – unless you have a distraction.

Coping with Sugar 'Dealers'

WEDDINGS, BIRTHDAYS, CHRISTENINGS

- **Choose one favourite food**. At a party, the table is generally loaded with different sweet foods – sponge cakes, iced biscuits, mini chocolate bars. If it's your celebration, allow yourself your *very* favourite food to eat. For example, if you love a particular type of chocolate cake, you can have it on the day. Make a big deal of it – make it your birthday cake with candles on it *but* remember you can't have any other sweet foods. At least this way, you can gauge how much you've eaten rather than totally losing track and giving in to your sugar desires.
- **Say 'no' to sweet gifts**. Chocolate is such an easy present to give someone so most of us receive at least one box on birthdays or at events like Christmas. If this is you, either say, 'That's really kind of you, but I'm trying not to eat them' and give them back. Or why not donate them to someone you know (for example, an elderly neighbour) or to a school tombola? If someone wants to buy you a sweet treat, ask for dried dates or figs, or even some luxury tropical-fruit mix. If you have to succumb to chocolate, make it dark chocolate with at least 70 per cent cocoa solids (try Green and Black's, which you can now buy in most supermarkets).

2. Family and Friends
The 'Dealers'
- **Keeping people happy.** We all want our family and friends to be happy, but sometimes this desire can play against us. If you're the family chef who always makes delicious desserts, you may feel you're letting people down if you tell them you're not going to be making treacle pudding anymore. Or perhaps you're the one who always finishes food on your plate because you're worried people will be upset if you don't.
- **The way you've always been 'seen'.** It's easy to get pigeonholed, whether you're the 'cuddly' mum, the grandma who's known for her sweet tooth or the friend who can always be relied upon to down plenty of drinks. We're all perceived a certain way by people in our lives, whether we're happy with that label or not.
- **Force of habit.** You make the same foods time and again – and people love you for it! If you don't make your special trifle, treacle pudding or steak and kidney pie, you may worry that people will be upset with you.
- Not wanting to be different. If your friends eat a certain way (for example, never eating breakfast or regular meals), you might feel tempted to do the same as them so you don't stand out.

Coping with Sugar 'Dealers'

How to Cope
- **Take control of mealtimes.** If you're the cook, the buck stops with you so technically you can change the way you and your family eat. We're not saying you have to convert everyone to a sugar-free diet, but you can make small changes to the food you cook without them even knowing. For example, changing normal rice to low-GI basmati, making a simple tomato pasta sauce instead of using sugar-laden bottled varieties or using Quorn as an occasional substitute to meat to help widen their palate.
- **Keep everyone happy – including you!** If you've always been known for your good desserts, there's no reason this should stop. Look at our recipe options in Chapter 15, or look in cookbooks for diabetics or people with Candida for other tempting sugar-free ideas. You'll soon see there's no need to forfeit taste. If they insist on eating their usual dessert, you will not feel so 'left out' if you make a sugar-free version for yourself (such as a cheesecake), wherever possible.
- **Send your guests home with tempting leftovers.** If it's a special occasion or a guest has brought a dessert with them to 'help you out', don't be tempted to keep any leftovers. You may tell yourself it's going straight in the bin, but chances are it won't … Instead, have a supply of paper plates or disposable containers ready to send food home with the guests.

- **Get them on your side**. Friends and family don't have to be your downfall – they could actually be your salvation. Put them in the picture as to what you're doing and how they could help you, and you'll almost certainly find your attempts to cut out sugar will be easier. Ask a close friend or relative to be your 'sugar buddy' whom you can call when you're tempted by sugar, feeling low or want to share your success of turning down some sweets or losing a few pounds.
- **Out of sight, out of mind**. There's nothing worse than someone tempting you with a treat you know you can't have. Ask family members to enjoy them in another room.

3. Girls' Nights Out
The 'Dealers'
- **Peer pressure**. You're on a girls' night out or a holiday with friends, and not only do you have that little voice inside you telling you to eat sweets, you also have your friends egging you on. Even if they're not encouraging you to eat sugary foods, the sight of them doing it can lead you astray.
- **Going out without eating**. When you're heading out for a night with the girls and your focus is on getting ready, it's easy to forget to eat – or at least to just grab some crisps or chocolate to keep you going. The same applies if you go to the pub or a bar straight after work.

How to Cope
- **Eat before you go out.** Invite friends to your place first so you're all in the same situation and they're less likely to end up going for a burger afterwards. Drinking on an empty stomach is never a good idea anyway, so filling up beforehand means you're less likely to be ill with a hangover the next day.
- **Always take snacks with you.** OK, so you've only got a small handbag. But how much room do a few nuts take up? This is especially important if you're going on a big night out where you may well be out for hours. If you end up not eating you will find yourself with low blood-sugar. For a bit of incentive, just think of that new outfit you want to buy and how much better you'd look in it just one size smaller …
- **Stockpile healthy options in your desk or work fridge.** If there's always something for you to eat at work, you'll have no need to go for those after work drinks on an empty stomach. Even if it's just an apple with some cheese or some crispbread with peanut butter, at least it'll be something to keep you ticking over.
- **Choose soft drinks with care.** If you're not drinking alcohol, you may spend the evening drinking cola, lemonade or even a sweetened water drink. But remember, lots of sweetened water drinks (such as Appletise) contain high levels of sugar. If you want flavoured water, ask for mineral water with a slice

of lemon, lime or orange (or all three!). Have water, soda (not tonic or diet tonic) or even unsweetened fruit juice as a mixer with spirits or wine, and avoid lemonades and other sugar-laden drinks.

4. Holidays
The 'Dealers'
- **Lack of routine.** This is one of the reasons holidays are so great – you don't have to do the things you normally would. But if you're trying to eat healthily, lack of routine can see your good intentions going out of the window. For example, if you're used to eating lunch at 12.30pm but there's nowhere to get it until 2pm, you could end up eating unhealthy snacks to keep your energy levels up.
- **Poor availability of healthy foods.** This depends on where you go. If you're in a country where they eat a lot of fresh fruit then you're likely to make better food choices than if you're somewhere where the staple diet is processed ready meals, nightly takeaways or even deep-fried Mars Bars!
- **'Go on – you're on holiday!'** We're not saying you shouldn't be enjoying the local cuisine or letting your hair down when it comes to special holiday foods. The trouble is, most of us go overboard. If it's a two-week holiday we'll generally eat for Britain, then we return to the UK and carry on indulging to mask our depression that the holiday's over. The net result? We

Coping with Sugar 'Dealers'

fall off the sugar wagon and stress about how we're going to get back on it again.

How to Cope
- **Take snacks with you**. Take stock ingredients with you in your luggage, such as nuts, dried fruit and crispbread. Your snack foods may be in plentiful supply at your destination – if you're going to the Mediterranean, for example, there will probably be a better choice of nuts in the shops than we have in the UK. But you may be going somewhere where the choice is limited – American foods, for instance, tend to be low-fat but very high in sugar so your 'normal' choice might actually be a bad choice in the States.
- **Be prepared for all eventualities**. We all know delays are as much a part of holidays as tummy bugs and sunburn. Don't forget to take plenty of snacks in your hand luggage to munch on at the airport in case this happens to you.
- **Ask for a 'special diet' meal when you book your plane ticket**. For example, you could ask for a fresh fruit platter, or a diabetic meal, which excludes sugars, syrups, jams, cakes and chocolate, unless they are diabetic forms. They are still likely to be sweet but unlikely to give you a sugar 'rush'.
- **Remember the carb and protein/dairy combo**. You can't always tell whether you're eating healthy or not-so-healthy foods when you're abroad. But try and

stick to the basic Sugar Addicts' Diet principle of always eating carbs with proteins. That way you'll help keep some kind of routine and, in doing so, maintain good blood-sugar levels to stop you falling off the wagon and gorging on sugar. So, for example, if the menu option is pepperoni or ham pizza and chips, have it with a salad and extra vegetable toppings, such as spinach and onions. These 'extras' will help reduce the GI and therefore the impact on your blood-sugar levels. Take this book with you (or copy Chapters 8 and 9) so you know which foods are carbs and which are protein/dairy.

5. Eating Out
The 'Dealers'
- **Sugary desserts**. If there are six desserts on the menu, chances are just one will be a healthy fruit option. And most of us want to let our hair down and enjoy something gooey and sugary as a treat once in a while.
- **Alcohol**. Let's face it – for most of us a meal out just doesn't feel the same without alcohol.
- **'Eat all you can' offers**. Restaurants usually offer these in slow periods (such as midweek lunchtimes) or in the knowledge you'll make up for it in drink purchases.
- **'Would you like fries with that?'** You went in thinking you'd just have a burger and you walked out

with a double burger with extra large fries and a bucket of cola. When someone asks you if you 'want fries with that?' how can you resist?
- **The 'go on' voice inside you.** You're out for a family barbecue, lunch with friends or a dinner with your partner. It's a special occasion and the voice inside you is saying, 'Go on – treat yourself!'

How to Cope
- **Don't skip savoury to go on to sweet.** You may think you'll save yourself some calories and be 'in credit' if you skip the main course and go straight onto the dessert. Don't do it – a carb and protein main is vital for blood-sugar control. If you only eat a sweet your blood-glucose levels will be all over the place and you may find yourself stuffing even more in to give yourself an energy boost. If you have a savoury meal, your body will be better able to cope with a mouthful of a sweet option afterwards.
- **Share a dessert.** People will often order a dessert 'to share' when they really want one themselves but can't admit it. Admit you want one, promise to share it with a friend and just enjoy your half of it! Choose something 'solid' like a cake or tart rather than something 'sloppy' like ice cream. That way you can cut it in half and know exactly how much you're eating, rather than saying you've had half when your eating partner has only managed to grab a spoonful!

- **Go overboard with the vegetables**. When your main course comes out, fill up on vegetables, whether it's extra side orders or ordering a salad. Or why not try a vegetable-based dish such as moussaka, risotto or a stir-fry? Vegetables are naturally low in sugar and will help stabilize your blood-sugar levels. When choosing from a salad bar, go for grated carrot, beetroot and sweetcorn to satisfy your need for a sweet taste. But avoid salad dressings apart from oil and vinegar – as well as being made with the wrong kind of fats (often hydrogenated), options like thousand island dressing or mayonnaise are generally *packed* full of sugars.
- **Choose alcohol wisely**. Alcohol is full of sugar, especially liqueurs, beers and alcopops. Go for wine (try a dry white wine spritzer with soda *not* lemonade) or vodka (with fizzy water or a small amount of unsweetened fruit juice, *not* tonic water). If you can't help yourself and know you're likely to binge, offer to be the 'designated driver' and stick to non-sugary, non-alcoholic drinks such as fizzy water with slices of lemon, lime or orange. Sounds boring, but imagine no hangover from alcohol *or* sugar.
- **If it doesn't look like meat, avoid it!** Avoid processed 'reconstituted' options such as burgers, hot dogs or sausages, which often have lots of sugar and salt in them. Go instead for burgers made from whole pieces of meat (often called 'chicken breast fillet'), lean fillets (with rind or fat cut off) or even vegetarian

Coping with Sugar 'Dealers'

options (though watch out for veggie options laden with fatty cheese or cream). At barbecues, avoid the burgers and sausages and go instead for chicken drumsticks (without the skin), veggie burgers or fish.

- **Eat any sweet treats S-L-O-W-L-Y**. If you've been sticking to the Sugar Addicts' Diet and feel your blood-sugar levels are now on an even keel, you may feel ready to allow yourself a sweet treat. Enjoy each spoonful at a time. That way you'll get pleasure from each small bit, rather than wolfing it down and wanting more. And always eat sweet foods with your main meal to prevent a blood-sugar 'spike'.
- **Entertain at home instead**. If someone suggests you go out, why not offer to cook instead? It's a chance to practise your culinary skills but it also means you can oversee ingredients so you know *exactly* what has gone into the meal. Meals don't have to be complicated (see some of our recipes in Chapter 15 for suggestions).
- **Help yourself to less**. If you're helping yourself to an 'eat as much as you can' menu, go up once and put on your plate about a quarter of what you'd normally be tempted to eat. If you can't help piling it high, use a side plate instead. For other restaurant meals, aim to leave half the course on your plate. If that sounds hard, as soon as you're halfway through, put your serviette on your plate so you won't be tempted to eat any more, or ask the waiter to remove your plate before others have finished.

- **Supersize tactics**. Some fast-food restaurants have announced plans to scrap 'supersizing' but until they do, what can you do? If you want something 'extra', go instead for one of their healthier options like a yoghurt, some milk, fruit or a portion of salad.

Restaurant Tips
- **Consider the cooking method**. Go for dishes that are grilled, boiled, poached, steamed or stir-fried, rather than deep-fried, breaded or with pastry (such as pies). If you can't tell from the menu how the food is cooked, ask the waiter or waitress. Steer away from rich and creamy dishes, and meals that contain lots of cheese, because these tend to be high in fat.
- **Italian**. When ordering pizza, choose lower-fat toppings, such as vegetables, ham, tuna and prawns, and avoid ground beef, pepperoni/salami and varieties loaded with different cheeses. If pasta is the dish of the day, try to choose a sauce based on tomatoes or vegetables, rather than cream.
- **Indian**. Avoid creamy curries, such as korma, passanda or massala, especially with fatty meats such as lamb. Go instead for tandoori or madras with chicken, prawns or vegetables. Choose plain rice and chapatti rather than pilau rice and naan.
- **Chinese**. Lower-fat options include steamed fish, chicken chop suey and Szechuan prawns, while anything with batter is best avoided. Sweet and sour

pork is usually battered (ask if you're not sure).
- **Thai**. Stick to stir-fried or steamed dishes containing chicken, fish or vegetables. Green and red curries contain coconut milk, which is high in saturated fat, so if you do choose a curry, leave some of the sauce.
- **Hamburger restaurants**. Some fast-food chains such as McDonald's are now offering healthier options. There are salads or vegetarian alternatives, such as Quorn burgers, for those who want fast-food without excessive fat and calories. If these aren't available, opt instead for a fillet (such as a chicken fillet) which is a proper cut of meat rather than a burger which is minced meat with extra fat.

6. Supermarket 'Sneaks'
The 'Dealers'
- **BOGOF**. No, we're not being rude – we're talking 'buy one, get one free'. Or three for the price of two. These offers are fine if they're for healthy foods such as chicken breasts or mixed nuts. But generally they're not. The offers are on products such as multi-packs of crisps, biscuits and other processed foods such as ready meals. They're often a good deal so they're hard to resist.
- **Sweets at the checkout**. You know what we mean – you've shopped like a saint, only to find that as you wait to pay, there are stacks of sweets just *pleading*

with you to buy them. Some people aren't swayed by these but if you're a sugar-lover, you probably are!
- **Sugary foods among healthy foods**. You can go to a supermarket with all the best intentions to keep away from sugary, processed foods, only to discover that they're lurking in aisles where you least expected to find them. For example, extra sugary muesli next to the porridge, or a sticky toffee apple in the fruit and veg section.
- **So-called 'healthy' ranges**. Many supermarkets have their own range of 'healthy' foods that you'd expect to be low in sugar. Right? Not necessarily. Many of these ranges are low in fat, calorie counted and salt-controlled, as well as avoiding artificial colours, flavour enhancers and preservatives where possible. But many are also high in sugar.

How to Cope
- **Beat them at their own game**. Supermarkets employ clever psychology to get you to buy more, and not necessarily foods that are good for you. For example, they place fruit and veg at the front of the store because it's bulky, which will encourage you to choose a trolley rather than a basket. Think to yourself, 'Do I really need a trolley, or am I just going to fill it with rubbish?' If you do take one, use the opportunity to pile it up with this fresh produce, rather than leaving loads of space for when you get near the biscuit aisle.

Coping with Sugar 'Dealers'

- **Beware of impulse purchases**. Certain shops are definitely worse than others when it comes to displaying tempting sweets at the checkout, so if you know you're likely to be tempted, try and go to a different shop. In a 2003 survey, the Food Commission found that Asda was the worst and Waitrose was the best, but it also found sweets at the tills of unexpected places such as Mothercare and pharmacies including Boots. If you can't avoid these shops, make sure you occupy yourself in some way when you get to the checkout. Maybe browse through one of the magazines they're also trying to get you to buy! Consumer psychologist Sue Keane advises speaking to the manager about moving these products. 'They're businesses and they'll do almost anything to keep customers happy.'
- **Shop online**. Online shopping services are now offered by lots of supermarkets including Sainsbury's, Tesco, Safeway, Iceland and Waitrose. This enables you to avoid queues and shop at your convenience (the middle of the night when the kids are asleep, for example). You're also less likely to be tempted by fancy packaging. The great thing is that for each product, they list the ingredients so you can see what has sugar in and what doesn't. Make a conventional list before you start and don't deviate from it – unless, of course, it's to buy something sugar-free you haven't tried before.

- **Make a list and stick to it**. We all know what happens when we shop without a list – we end up buying what we *didn't* need, like sweets we saw advertised on television, and arrive home without key essentials. Make a list and don't waver from it. Also, experts say that if we make a list with the store's layout in mind, we're less likely to be tempted by things we don't need.
- **Keep to the outside of the supermarket**. Among the wide array of tactics used by supermarkets to get you to buy more is putting all the essentials – milk, bread, meat and fresh produce – on the perimeter of the store. The layout encourages you to go up and down the aisles where expensive – and generally sugary and processed – foods are kept. So if you keep to the outside as much as possible, you'll avoid temptation, as well as saving yourself some money. If you can't handle temptation, don't even go there!
- **Never shop on an empty stomach**. It's an age-old suggestion, but it really does make a difference, especially if you're going to a supermarket where they're baking bread and your weakness just happens to be for fresh white loaves … Also, avoid buying food to eat on the way home. Instead, buy something healthy you know you can quickly prepare for yourself once you get there.
- **Listen to music while you shop**. Studies have shown that slow music makes shoppers linger over their

shopping. The more you linger, the more money you're likely to spend. And the longer you're in the supermarket, the more tempted you may be to buy sugary foods. Wear a personal stereo playing moderate to fast music and you're likely to shop quicker.
- **Watch out for sugars**. We assume many of these must be healthy 'by association' – if a fruit yoghurt is next to a plain yoghurt, it must be healthy, right? Not necessarily – this is where your label-reading skills come in. Don't ever assume things are healthy because of where they are in the supermarket. Don't be complacent about a supermarket's 'healthy' range – use your eyes! Use your 'sugar detective' skills to see if it's a food you really want to buy. Look at Chapter 7 to remind yourself of the names sugar often goes under.

7. Manufacturers and Advertisers
The 'Dealers'
- **New products**. When a new sweet food is advertised, are you straight down the shops trying to buy it? If this is you, it's not a sign of weakness. You're living proof of how powerful advertising can be.
- **Adverts aimed at children**. Kids are watching more television than ever before, and 99 per cent of the foods advertised are high in fat, sugar and salt. They watch the adverts, then come to you pleading for these products to be put on your shopping list.

- **Adverts aimed at adults**. It's not just kids who fall for these ads. After all, adults have the greatest spending power. Millions of pounds are spent each year on consumer surveys to work out what we want to buy and why, and advertising campaigns to get us to part with our money. Some ads are annoying, lots are memorable and too many encourage us to buy foods we know we probably shouldn't.
- **Vending machines with 'eat me' messages**. We swear vending machines have a magnet in them that pulls sugar-lovers to them. You need a will of steel to walk past one without getting your money out.

How to Cope

- **Channel surf away from tempting ads**. If you know the adverts are coming up (the little thing in the corner!) then switch to a channel that doesn't have ads. Or get up during the break and walk around.
- **Video your favourite programmes**. If your favourite shows are on commercial channels and you find ads hard to resist, video them so you can fast forward through the adverts. It's hard to be tempted when the commercials are playing at 64 times the speed!
- **Distract kids during ad breaks**. This isn't always easy – you could find yourself running in and out of the room every 10 minutes or so. But if you can do it, each time the ads come on have something else to take

their attention away from the screen. For example, a snack to be collected from the kitchen, something that needs fetching from upstairs or just a conversation about what they've been watching or what's been happening at school.
- **Don't give vending machines a look-in**. Have snacks ready to cope with those 'vending machine moments' (usually when a colleague says they're going and would you like anything …). Know what your weaknesses are. If you miss opening a pack of something savoury, have a packet snack such as pretzels or some nuts ready, or a sweet fruit bar or yoghurt-coated pineapple chunks (see 'Good Shop-bought Options' in Chapter 11). Encourage your workplace to put some healthy options in their vending machine, or change to a 'green' one.
- **Beware of 'buzzwords'**. There are certain words we automatically assume mean a food is sugar-free, like 'organic', 'all natural', 'healthy' or 'wholewheat.' This isn't necessarily the case – after all, you can have organic sugar but it's *still* sugar! Just keep your eyes peeled.

8. That's Entertainment
The 'Dealers'
- **Bad food EVERYWHERE!** The options for someone trying to cut down on sugar are generally very limited. Most shelf space is dedicated to

SUGAR ADDICTS' DIET

processed foods that are generally high in fat, sugar and additives like colourings.

- **The dreaded pick 'n' mix stall.** Pick 'n' mix has been around for years but stalls selling it are now popping up in places you'd least expect, such as in clothes shops. The problem is that it's up to you to decide how much to buy, and when you're faced with all that choice, you are bound to pile too much into the bag. Try and avoid the stall completely, but if you can't, take as few sweets as you can in one hand and buy just those. If any topple off, you're being too greedy.
- **Going to the cinema.** If you haven't got a bucket of toffee popcorn, an extra large drink and a family pack of sweets, it doesn't feel like a real trip to the cinema. The whole movie experience seems to lend itself to sitting there eating while you get engrossed in a film. Take your own food – Nicki cuts up apples, strawberries, pears and oranges and puts them in a plastic sandwich bag to chomp on while she's there. Another good tactic is to take your own homemade popcorn. Ask for an empty popcorn box while you're there and put your own popcorn in it – this is especially good if you've got kids who don't want to feel 'left out'. Another option is to buy Popz Popping Corn from the supermarket (either natural or salted but not the sugared varieties). It comes in a popcorn-style box, ready to put in the microwave for 'no-fuss' popcorn.

Coping with Sugar 'Dealers'

- **Waiting in the petrol-station queue**. You're standing behind three people while you wait to pay, and alongside you are rows and rows of sweets. It's temptation all the way, right up until you pay. And it's generally at that point that you throw in a bar of chocolate as the amount is being run up.

How to Cope
- **Pop a breath freshener in your mouth**. Just as sweets taste horrible if you've just brushed your teeth, they're similarly unappealing if you use one of those breath fresheners that dissolve on your tongue. When you sense a tempting sugar moment ahead – such as standing in a petrol station queue or during half time at a football match – pop one in your mouth.
- **Pick 'n' mix substitutes**. Take your own pick 'n' mix of dried tropical fruit in a paper bag. These mixes often include papaya, pineapple, mango, apricots, peaches and pears so are naturally sweet, and they're dried so they have a great texture as your teeth sink into them. If you have to choose sweets from the pick 'n' mix, go for boiled sweets and make sure you suck them so they're long-lasting, or chocolate nuts and raisins.
- **Petrol station**. If you know you're going to be distracted by the sweets, buy a magazine or paper so you can read it while you're in the queue as a form of distraction.

SUGAR ADDICTS' DIET

- **Buy a bottle of water**. People often mistake being slightly thirsty for being hungry or peckish. This is more likely to strike you if you've been somewhere dehydrating such as on a car journey or in a hot cinema. Have a bottle of water to hand and take a good gulp when you think you're feeling hungry. You'll probably find you feel a lot better.
- **Go for savoury snacks**. If the choice is between salty savoury snacks or sweets, you can't win! We're not saying lots of salt is great, because it isn't. But if you're trying to get away from craving sugar, you're better off having a bit of salted popcorn or some tortilla chips when you go to the cinema. Go for extra spicy tortilla chips as you're likely to eat these more slowly.
- **Arrive late**. We're not telling you to miss the start of the film, but often there's at least 15 minutes or so of adverts to go through before you see the movie you paid to watch. Arrive early and you'll be in plenty of time to be tempted by the sweets, adverts for fatty, sugary foods and other people rustling pick 'n' mix bags. Arrive just as the film is starting and you'll miss your chance to be tempted. Book ahead and you'll have no excuses!

9. The Boredom Factor
The 'Dealers'
- **Too much time on your hands**. Life always seems to be about extremes – you're either running around like a headless chicken, or you're climbing the walls with boredom. Those times when you've nothing to do can be dangerous when it comes to eating the wrong foods.
- **Munching without realizing**. Whether transfixed on your favourite soap, having a coffee break with a magazine or on a shopping trip, so many of us munch away without even realizing what we're doing. Before we know it, we've eaten a whole packet of chocolate raisins to ourselves ...
- **Giving yourself a hard time**. When you're sitting alone without anyone around to act as the 'voice of reason', it's all too easy to be dragged down by negative thoughts about yourself. Whether it's 'I'm ugly', 'I'm so fat' or 'I'm useless', that phrase can be so destructive that the only way you can feel better is to eat something comforting.

How to Cope
- **Keep your hands busy**. If you're used to mindlessly munching as you watch television then it's time to give your hands something else to do instead. Try squeezing a stress ball or some 'silly putty'. If you can concentrate on your hands instead of the television,

SUGAR ADDICTS' DIET

try playing cards or doing some sewing or painting (a picture or your nails!).
- **Don't eat on the move**. If you're shopping, don't allow yourself to eat on the move – eating is strictly for when you're sitting down in a café or restaurant.
- **Put obstacles in your way**. By this we mean putting obstacles in the way of you getting to unhealthy food. For example, stash sweets in the freezer to keep temptation at bay. This works well for jelly sweets (not so great for chocolate, which tastes infinitely better when it's been frozen!). Thawing them will give you time to consider whether you really want them.
- **Brush your teeth**. When you have a sugar craving, brush your teeth. This will make most sweets taste terrible.
- **Sort your house out**. Get busy. Make a list of small jobs in the house that need doing and, when you're feeling bored, do one of those jobs instead of eating sugar. Not only will you be avoiding sugar – you'll also be getting tasks done that you've probably been putting off for ages.
- **Have a snooze**. If your blood-sugar levels aren't properly balanced and you're in a sugar 'dip', you might well feel tired. Instead of reaching for sugar as a pick-me-up, have a 10-minute power nap instead, followed by a protein and carb snack when you wake to help normalize blood-glucose levels.

- **Think 'thin'**. If your goal is weight loss, hang up an outfit from your 'thin wardrobe' in your living room to remind you of your aim. There's no point leaving it in your bedroom – put it somewhere highly visible as a constant reminder. And tell friends and family why it's there so they can help you to keep on track.
- **Have a mantra**. 'A what?' we hear you say. A mantra is a word or phrase that you say to yourself to help you feel positive. If you've been stuck with a negative phrase all your life, now is the time to replace it with a positive one. Each time you feel the negative thoughts coming in, have a positive phrase ready. Create it by thinking the exact opposite of your negative one. For example, instead of 'I'm ugly', say to yourself 'I'm beautiful and fantastic'; instead of 'I'm so fat' say 'I'm popular and I love myself as much as others love me'. You may laugh the first time you say it, but you'll be surprised at how quickly you'll start to feel empowered by it.

10. Being a Parent
The 'Dealers'
- **Finishing off the kids' food**. If they don't eat it, it's so easy to end up eating it for them. There's also the common ploy of buying a packet of sweets 'for them' as a way of buying them for yourself ...
- **Falling for the hype**. Many adverts for children's foods are aimed at parents. Some products claim to

have health benefits (such as extra calcium) that tug on the heart strings and make parents feel guilty if they don't buy them. Any parent will tell you these can be hard to resist.
- **Pester power**. Bright packaging and food strategically placed so it's within reach of tiny grabbing fingers mean a shopping trip with kids can turn into an all-out battle of wills.
- **Handling doting relatives**. Grandparents will often say it's their job to 'spoil the grandchildren'. In the past, when kids were more active, the occasional bar of chocolate, packet of sweets or can of drink was no problem. Now our kids are fatter than they've ever been and their love of sugar isn't helping. But try telling that to grandparents – they just want to spread a little happiness!

How to Cope
- **Squirt the washing-up liquid**. When the kids have left the table and you're tempted to eat the leftovers, get the washing-up liquid and squirt it all over the plate. Even if you're not washing up straight away, it will stop you picking at the food. A perfect, foul-tasting deterrent!
- **Shop without the kids**. If you've ever shopped with a kid, you'll know the meaning of 'pester power'. They know what they want and they'll try their hardest to get it. It doesn't help that supermarkets place items

Coping with Sugar 'Dealers'

that will appeal to kids, such as sweets, at their eye level so it's almost impossible for you to prevent it. If you have to take them with you, allow them one special item each *and no more*!

- **Leave your partner at home**. OK, we know they're not kids, but sometimes it feels like they are! Research suggests that when women shop with their partners, they tend to spend more money and are more likely to try out new items. It also suggests men tend to get so bored that they buy the first item that catches their eye, rather than concentrating on buying the most appropriate food. Leave him at home and do your shopping *your* way!
- **Re-educating grandparents**. A visit to the grandparents means raiding the biscuit tin or finding the sweets they've got in especially. But these don't have to be kept in quantity – either take these treats to grandparents yourself (so at least you know what they're having) and only provide enough for the one or two treats they're allowed. The more there are, the more likely grandparents will be to 'give in' and let kids have them all. Let kids know, too, that they're not going to be able to do any 'arm-twisting' to get more food. Help grandparents understand that the kids won't love them any less if they withhold unhealthy foods. Teach them to look at other ways of providing a 'treat', such as taking them to places or watching videos with them.
- **'Concealing' healthy food**. Sometimes kids just won't

eat healthy food, no matter what you do. Studies show that many parents don't bother buying healthy foods because it'll be a waste of money if their kids refuse to eat them. Why not try and 'hide' some healthy things in their food without them realizing? For example, if you make a Bolognaise sauce, finely grate some carrot into it, which will help to bulk it up (so it'll go further) and make it healthier. Or put some carrot juice into their orange juice, or mix orange juice with their squash as you try and 'wean' them off it.

- **Find good alternatives to foods they'd normally go for**. If you're making a sandwich where you'd normally use mayonnaise (such as tuna mayo), use plain yoghurt with a bit of low-fat cream cheese (such as Philadelphia Light).
- **Sip while they're eating**. While you're cooking for yourself and the kids, make yourself a drink to sip (like a tea or half and half fruit juice). Sip it while they're eating and carry on sipping until all the food is out of the way. That way you're still getting some taste pleasures without having to finish off their food.
- **Be inspired by your children**. If your problem is your own sugar addiction (rather than your children's), use your kids as inspiration for helping yourself. Think of all the things you'll be able to do with them now if you lose weight or stop feeling so sluggish, and all the things you'll be able to do in the future if you're fit and healthy for them as they grow up.

Part 3:

Break Your Sugar Addiction in Three Weeks

13

The 21-day Plan

This chapter takes you, step by step, through our 21-day plan. There are five stages, from preparing for the diet right through to what to do when the three weeks are over. We will be with you at every step as you learn to control your sugar addiction and start eating healthily.

STAGE 1: PREPARING FOR THE DIET

You wouldn't throw a party or go on holiday without preparing, would you? So why would you just launch into a diet without getting a few important things in place first? Before you begin Stage 2 – 'Starting the Diet' (page 252) – you should have some emotional and practical 'helpers' in place. These are:

- keeping a diary
- getting to know the 21-day meal plan
- stocking up on food for the plan

This will ensure nothing gets in the way of your new, healthier eating plan. You can do this preparation in a day, or over several days if it suits you better. You could even do it a week before you start Stage 2 – the important thing is actually doing the preparation so you get things ready for the diet itself.

Start to Keep a Diary
Why: This will help you to understand your triggers for eating, what you're eating, and where the sugar is in your diet.

As we explain in Chapter 3, a diary can really help you see what you eat, how you eat (such as on the run, always out of packets!) and when you eat (such as when you're stressed, tired or even happy). By being more aware of these things, you can start to see the messages your body is giving you about your relationship with food. For example, it could be that you have symptoms of poor blood-sugar control, but you may be unaware of them until you write them down. A diary can also help you be more honest with yourself – if you write it down, it's less easy to forget those chips you ate off a friend's plate or those five jelly babies you've managed to tell yourself you didn't scoff!

Action
- **Get your diary ready**. Either take a copy of the diary page in Chapter 3 or get an exercise book or notebook and draw out the grids yourself. Choose a method you know is convenient for you – there's no point in having your diary in a hardback A4 book if you only ever carry

a handbag around. Remember, you'll be filling it in at various points during the day so it's got to be handy.
- **What to write**. Each time you eat, make a note of the time ('Time of day'), what you ate (Food/Drink), how it made you feel ('Physical symptoms' and 'How you're feeling') and other relevant factors, such as whether you ate in a rush or had a cold or other illness. It's also important to write down how you feel after eating, if the food has an ill effect. For example, you may feel sick after eating sugar.
- **See it as a help, not a hindrance**. Having to fill in a diary each time you eat something can sound like a real drag. But it's a great tool that can really help boost your chances of success on the Sugar Addicts' Diet.
- **Put your goals in**. Your diary is a tool to help you understand how and why you eat the way you do. It can also be there to help motivate you. As well as writing your first entry on day one, write down what your goals are. In other words, what you'd like to get out of the diet. These goals can be as big or small as you want – a mixture is good to help you feel motivated when you achieve the smaller ones and to encourage you to carry on towards the bigger ones. Your goals might be to lose weight, feel healthier, have a better self-image, get a boyfriend or drop a dress size. Or they may be doing a weekly exercise class, fitting into the jeans you bought five years ago,

having better skin, walking down the biscuit aisle of the supermarket without stopping or managing to say 'no' when someone offers you sweets With each day of the plan, refer back to this list to tick things off as and when you achieve them, and to remind yourself why you're doing the diet!

- *Relevant chapter: Chapter 3, page 35*

Nicki's Tips

You don't have to write pages and pages in your diary. If you're no wordsmith, just use single words to describe how you feel. A simple 'bloated' or 'depressed' says just as much as a long sentence!

Get to Know the Meal Plan
Why: This is to help you feel comfortable with 'new' foods.

The purpose of this is to get you thinking about food in a different way. It might sound strange but this diet could be totally different to the one you're eating at the moment and it may take some getting used to. Getting to know the meal plan is essentially 'getting your head round it'. Think of this as being a bit like reading a holiday brochure and working out what's what before you go ahead and book it.

The 21-day Plan

Action

- **Find the foods you like.** You might want to go through with a pen or pencil and put a tick next to the ones you like, a cross next to the ones you definitely don't and a question mark next to the ones you'd like to try. When it comes to health, a wide variety of foods is best.
- **'Mix and match' your meals.** The meal plan is for 21 days. This means you can follow it for 21 days without having to really think about it (other than buying and preparing it, of course!). But we're not saying you have to eat it in order from day 1 through to day 21, or even eat everything on it. For example, you could eat the snacks from day 2 instead of those in day 1. It's interchangeable so do it in whatever order suits you best. You will need to adapt the shopping list on pages 242–51 to reflect your meal choices.
- **Don't panic if there's lots you don't like.** There may be foods on the plan that don't agree with you or you simply don't like. It's best to have variety in your diet because different foods provide different nutrients, which is why we've included a wide range of options. But if you only find, say, one breakfast, three snacks and four lunches and dinners you like, then stick with those. There'll be plenty of time for you to try new things as the days or weeks go by. You can gradually become inventive, using the 'foods to eat/foods to avoid' lists to discover your own meal options.

- *Relevant chapter: Chapter 14, page 285*

Say Goodbye to 'Autopilot' Shopping
Why: This is to help you shop differently rather than on 'autopilot'.

Going to the supermarket is something you could probably do with your eyes shut – you know what shelves your favourite foods are on and in which aisle the best snacks are found. But soon you're going to have to shop with fresh eyes, possibly looking at foods you've never bought before – maybe never even heard of. By reading this book and looking at the hints, tips and advice on different foods, you'll start to gain more confidence in trying new things. But that's in the future – here's some advice on how to shop now.

Action
- **Make a list.** Take a look at the weekly shopping list, below. This lists the ingredients you will need to prepare all the meals in the 21-day plan.
- **Buy for at least a week.** You may already be an organized shopper (especially if you have a family to cater for) but if you're not, now's a good time to start. The reason? If you have healthy foods available at home, rather than letting them run out, you'll be less tempted by unhealthy foods or snacks. For example, if you run out of popcorn or nuts to munch at work, you might end up making a trip to the vending machine.

- **Don't kick out your old foods – yet!** At the moment, you'll still have your 'old' foods such as biscuits, sweets and cakes in your cupboard, and at this stage we're not asking you to kick them out. On day 15, it's going to be a case of 'out with the old and in with the new'. Until then, you can still enjoy the occasional sugary treat, but try and limit it to once a day. And always eat it with a meal, rather than on its own.
- *Relevant chapter: Chapter 14, page 285*

Weekly Shopping List for the 21-day Plan
These are the ingredients you will need to make the meals suggested in the 21-day plan. Please note that some of the recipes serve two or even four people. In week 1, you may find your shopping bill is higher than in weeks 2 and 3. This is because you'll be buying lots of basics, such as olive oil. Don't panic – these should last you for the entire plan, and even beyond. In some cases, you may find it easier and more economical to bulk buy in week 1 to last you in the coming weeks – for example, value packs of tinned sweetcorn and tomatoes.

Remember – these are the basics for the recipes. You may decide to buy even more fruit and veg for your snacks, so don't forget to add these to your shopping list.

SUGAR ADDICTS' DIET

WEEK 1
Bakery

- 1 loaf of grainy bread (e.g. Vogels)
- 1 loaf of rye bread
- 1 packet of Ryvita
- 1 multigrain roll
- 2 round wholemeal pitta breads (or 1 large one)

Groceries

- 8 corn tortillas (or 12 taco shells)
- 1 bottle of vanilla essence
- 2 litres of orange juice
- 1 packet of whole sweet almonds (100g)
- 1 jar of peanut butter
- 1 packet of sultanas (500g)
- 1 packet of dried apricots
- 1 packet of mixed nuts (300g)
- 1 packet of cashew nuts (150g)
- 1 packet of porridge (1kg)
- 1 packet of egg noodles (500g)
- 1 packet of basmati rice (1kg)
- 1 packet of fettuccini pasta (500g)
- 1 packet of spaghetti (500g)
- 2 cans of tomatoes (400g)
- 1 tube of tomato purée
- 1 can of red kidney beans (400g)
- 1 can of sugar-free baked beans (400g)

The 21-day Plan

1 can of tuna (200g)

1 small can of sweetcorn (350g)

1 medium jar of Marmite (250g)

1 jar of Dijon mustard

1 bottle of cider vinegar

1 bottle of balsamic vinegar

1 bottle of olive oil (500ml)

1 bottle of unsweetened soy sauce (150ml)

Chilli powder

Curry powder

Ground cinnamon

Dairy and fresh protein

300ml skimmed/semi-skimmed milk *per day*

1 large tub of plain yoghurt (500g)

Edam cheese (200g)

6 eggs

1 tub of reduced-fat houmous

Quorn mince (400g)

Sliced ham or Quorn 'ham' (250g)

1 tuna steak

2 skinned chicken breasts

1 roasting chicken (for Sunday lunch)

1 tub of low-fat cream cheese (e.g. Light Philadelphia) (200g)

1 carton of New Covent Garden soup

Low-fat margarine (e.g. Olivio or Pure with Sunflower)

SUGAR ADDICTS' DIET

Fresh fruit and vegetables

2 carrots

3 red peppers

1 green pepper

1 punnet of cherry tomatoes (250g)

2 sweet potatoes (400g)

4 medium-sized potatoes

Baby new potatoes (500g)

Button mushrooms (50g)

1 cauliflower

4 medium onions

1 bulb of garlic

1 packet of chives – chop it all and freeze excess for week 3

1 large lettuce

1 large cucumber

1 banana

1 pear

2 apples

1 melon

3 plums

1 bunch of grapes

Strawberries (100g)

Raspberries (50g)

Blueberries (50g)

Vegetables for roast dinner – e.g. 1 large broccoli, 4 carrots, baby new potatoes

Week 2

You should have enough of the following left over from last week so shouldn't have to buy any more at the moment:

'Basics'
- Whole sweet almonds
- Peanut butter
- Sultanas
- Mixed nuts
- Cashew nuts
- Porridge
- Marmite
- Basmati rice
- Dijon mustard
- Olive oil
- Tomato purée
- Cider vinegar
- Balsamic vinegar
- Vanilla essence
- Ground cinnamon
- Low-fat margarine
- Dried apricots
- Soy sauce

SUGAR ADDICTS' DIET

Things to buy:
Bakery

- 1 loaf of grainy bread (e.g. Vogels)
- 1 multigrain roll
- 1 packet of Ryvita

Groceries

- 2 litres of orange juice
- 1 pack of red or brown lentils (500g)
- 1 litre apple/pineapple juice
- 1 can of sugar-free baked beans (400g)
- 1 packet of sesame seeds
- 1 packet of macaroni (500g)
- 1 large can of tuna (200g)
- 1 small can of tuna (100g)
- 1 can of tomatoes (400g)
- 1 small can of sweetcorn (350g)

Dairy and fresh protein

- 300ml skimmed/semi-skimmed milk *per day*
- 1 tub of low-fat cream cheese (e.g. Light Philadelphia) (200g)
- 6 eggs
- Lean meat of choice (for roast dinner) – e.g. one lean chop per person
- Frozen prawns (400g) – will provide enough for next week
- Mozzarella cheese (45g)
- 1 packet of Edam cheese (200g) – if none is left from last week
- Lean minced beef (225g)
- 4 skinned chicken breasts

The 21-day Plan

2 salmon steaks (100g each)

1 large tub of plain yoghurt (500g)

1 packet of lean grilled bacon

1 carton of New Covent Garden soup

1 tub of low-fat cottage cheese (125g)

Fruit and vegetables

1 packet of dried apricots

1 packet of dried prunes

3 apples

1 can of pineapple in juice (200g)

1 packet of cooked beetroot (250g) – will provide enough for next week

Strawberries (100g)

Raspberries (200g)

Blueberries (50g)

2 peaches

2 pears

1 bunch of grapes

1 packet of fresh basil

1 punnet of cherry tomatoes (250g)

1 large lettuce

1 large cucumber

1 corn on the cob

2 medium carrots

3 medium onions

1 green pepper

1 medium courgette

1 bulb of garlic

SUGAR ADDICTS' DIET

1 large broccoli

1 packet of frozen spinach (1kg)

2 sweet potatoes (400g)

Baby new potatoes (500g)

1 packet of mangetout beans – will also do for Monday's dinner in week 3

1 leek (50g)

1 packet of fresh sage (or dried, if not available)

1 packet of fresh parsley – chop it all and freeze excess for week 3

Vegetables for roast dinner – e.g. 1 large broccoli, 4 carrots, baby new potatoes

Week 3

You should still have plenty of the basic ingredients mentioned in week 2's list, but double-check to make sure you're not going to run out as we'll be using most of them again in Week 3:

'Basics'

Whole sweet almonds

Peanut butter

Sultanas

Mixed nuts

Cashew nuts

Porridge

Marmite

Basmati rice

Dijon mustard

The 21-day Plan

Olive oil
Tomato purée
Cider vinegar
Balsamic vinegar
Vanilla essence
Ground cinnamon
Low-fat margarine
Dried apricots
Soy sauce

Things to buy:
Bakery

1 loaf of grainy bread (e.g. Vogels)
2 round wholemeal pitta breads (or 1 large one)
1 loaf of pumpernickel bread

Groceries

Carob powder
2 litres of orange juice
1 litre unsweetened apple juice
1 bottle of unsweetened chilli sauce
4 corn tortillas (or 6 taco shells)
1 small can of sweetcorn (350g)
3 cans of tomatoes (400g)
1 packet of lasagne pasta sheets (250g)
1 small bag of wholemeal flour
1 packet of egg noodles (500g)
2 tbsp of black pitted olives

SUGAR ADDICTS' DIET

1 tub of gravy granules
Dried oregano

Dairy and fresh protein

300ml skimmed/semi-skimmed milk *per day*
1 large tub of plain yoghurt (500g)
Brie cheese (50g)
Feta cheese (60g)
1 packet of Edam cheese (200g)
Sliced smoked salmon (100g)
1 tub of low-fat cream cheese (e.g. Philadelphia Light) (200g)
8 eggs
1 packet of turkey ham (100g)
1 small can of tuna (100g)
2 cod fillets (around 100g each)
Lean meat of choice for roast dinner (e.g. roasting turkey)
Quorn mince (200g)
Quorn sausages (4)

Fresh fruit and veg

1 bunch of grapes
1 packet of fresh dill
2 pears
1 peach
5 apples
1 large cucumber

The 21-day Plan

- 1 large lettuce
- Mushrooms (450g)
- 6 medium onions
- 2 red peppers
- 1 yellow pepper
- 3 green peppers
- Baby new potatoes (500g)
- 6 small potatoes for baking (200g)
- 1 sweet potato
- 1 small cauliflower
- 3 medium courgettes
- Mango (100g)
- Strawberries (200g)
- 1 punnet of cherry tomatoes (250g)
- 3 medium carrots
- 1 small aubergine
- 2 spring onions
- 4 fresh apricots
- 2cm length of root ginger
- Bean sprouts (100g)
- Vegetables for roast dinner – e.g. 1 large broccoli, 4 carrots, baby new potatoes

> ### Nicki's Tips
>
> *If you're not going to be using much of it in any given week, put your loaf of bread (e.g. rye bread) in the freezer and take out a slice as and when you need it. That way, none will go to waste. Do the same with pitta breads.*
>
> *If a recipe says 'use a quarter of an onion', chop up the whole onion and put it in the freezer in a freezer bag. That way, you don't waste any and you can just grab a handful when you need it for a recipe in the future.*

STAGE 2: STARTING THE DIET

Days 1–6 are about starting the 21-day eating plan. As we've just said, it may be that you pick and choose the meals you like, or you might prefer to go through each day as it comes. Either way, for the next six days we're going to be explaining exactly why these parts of the diet – such as always eating breakfast or taking some exercise – are so important when it comes to giving up sugar. However, don't expect to see 'give up sugar' in this section. That doesn't come until day 18.

The 21-day Plan

Day 1: Have a Proper Breakfast
Why: This is to try and get you to see breakfast as an important part of your daily routine.

'Breaking the fast' is essential to getting blood-sugar levels on an even keel. It's no coincidence that the old saying suggests you should 'Breakfast like a king'. Start the day without it and you'll find yourself reaching for something sugary mid-morning and your whole eating plan will go awry.

Action
- **Don't just think 'toast'.** The plan incorporates some good breakfast options. But it's important to know breakfast doesn't have to be conventional. If you'd rather have a chicken sandwich or some of last night's leftovers then go for it. The point is to stick with a carbohydrate and protein combination – exactly what that consists of is up to you.
- **Other breakfast suggestions.** There are lots of breakfast suggestions in the 'Eat Breakfast' section of Chapter 9, so if there aren't any you fancy in the 21-day plan, take a look here for some more ideas.
- **Can't stand the thought of breakfast?** Lots of people can't stomach eating in the morning. But we can't stress how important it is to try and have at least something. It can be liquid rather than solid, like a smoothie, so don't panic.

- **Write in your diary.** As well as making a note of what you're eating and when, don't forget to describe how it makes you feel, too.
- *Relevant chapter: Chapter 9, page 145*

Nicki's Tips

If you're one of those people who says they haven't got time for breakfast, perhaps you're overcomplicating it. Don't – there are plenty of sugar-free options that are in the box and ready to be put into the bowl, like Shredded Wheat.

Put dried fruits such as sultanas together with nuts and seeds in a pot so they're ready-mixed for you to spoon into your cereal.

Day 2: Eat Three Meals a Day

Why: Three meals with protein and carb will help stabilize blood-sugar levels and give you a feeling of 'fullness' that should tide you over from one meal to the next.

It may be that you're not used to eating regular meals – so many of us who've tried to diet will have skipped meals to save ourselves some calories. But missing out on meals makes your body go into starvation mode, which lowers your metabolic rate and means you won't

The 21-day Plan

burn up as many calories. If you feel like you've eaten properly, you'll also be less likely to stray towards fast-fix sweet foods. Eat three meals a day of the right kinds of foods and you'll keep your body ticking over nicely.

Action
- **Choose easy options**. If you know you've got a busy week ahead, don't make life difficult for yourself by going for options that need lots of preparation. Try quick and easy meals (such as jacket potatoes or pasta) instead. Leave more time-consuming options, such as trying out new recipes, for when you are less busy.
- **Cook in 'batches'**. Cooking more than you need may have been a temptation to eat too much in the past. But now you can use it to your advantage. Cook extra food, such as Bolognaise sauce, and put it in the freezer for another day. That way, if you are following each day of the plan, you'll have it to eat the following week without having to cook it from scratch.
- **Stick with foods you like**. We want you to stick with this diet because we know it works! But if you're not eating foods you like, you might easily fall off the wagon. In stage 1 we asked you to find the foods you like. If you're already in need of some more inspiration when it comes to options, look at Chapter 8 ('What to Eat'), Chapter 9 ('How to Eat', section on 'Eat the Right Carbs with Protein') and Chapter 11 (Hints and Tips for Giving up').

- ***Relevant chapter:*** *Chapter 8, page 119*

Nicki's Tip

If the thought of planning so many different meals seems a bit daunting, make things easier for yourself by eating the same breakfast each or every other day. That way you only have to use your brainpower on lunch and dinner!

Day 3: Learn Smart Snacking
Why: This is to show you that snacks don't have to be bad – if they're the right foods, they can help to keep your blood-sugar on an even keel all day long.
It's when you start getting hungry that you'll find your body craving a 'lift' from sugar. Snack properly and this doesn't need to happen!

Action
- **Snacks for your lifestyle.** Work out what snacks will best fit in with your lifestyle – for example, if you're at home during the weekend, your snacks can be more complicated than if you're out and about and need something more 'instant'.
- **Save food from the night before.** If you've got a little bit of your main meal left over, put it in a storage box

The 21-day Plan

in the fridge and have it as one of your snacks the next day. A bit of spaghetti Bolognaise or some of last night's chicken breast on a crispbread with a bit of salad are good protein and carbohydrate snack options that should help keep your blood-sugar steady.
- **Shopping for snacks**. If you're after a snack you can just buy off the shelf without having to prepare yourself, look at our list in Chapter 11 in 'Good Shop-bought Options'.
- *Relevant chapter: Chapter 9, page 145*

Day 4: Discover New Drinks
Why: To keep you hydrated throughout the day and ensure your body functions properly.
Unfortunately we don't mean alcoholic drinks! But you'll soon see that hydrating (having more fluids such as water) can make you feel far better than alcohol does – and with a longer-lasting effect. As you'll see from Chapter 8, water is essential for keeping the body working properly. It's vital for metabolism and for flushing out toxins. Giving your body at least 8–10 glasses of water a day helps keep you healthy and less groggy (with the added benefit of helping your skin to be healthy).

Action
- **Discover interesting new drinks**. That way you can start to incorporate more water into your daily routine.

And remember – small steps count. Even one mug of herb tea can start you on your path to better hydration.
- *Relevant chapter: Chapter 8, page 119*

> ### Nicki's Tip
>
> *If you're not used to drinking water, don't expect to be able to 'up' the levels right away. One glass at a time is a real achievement if you're starting off from nothing or making the switch from sugary canned drinks or coffee. Had one glass today? Pat yourself on the back and aim for two tomorrow, three the next and so on.*

Day 5: Eat Before Bed
Why: If you're hungry before you hit the sack, your blood-sugar levels will be low and you won't sleep properly.

Eat the right foods before bed and you'll stabilize blood-sugar and possibly even boost serotonin levels, helping you to sleep. Try to eat your bedtime snack around an hour before bedtime so the nutrients in the food can take effect without your meal sitting heavily in your stomach.

Action
- **Choose a satisfying snack.** A slow-release carbohydrate food like a small jacket potato, muesli or

porridge eaten an hour before bed is a good option. It has the double benefit of aiding sleep and levelling out blood-sugar so you won't wake in the night hungry – and on the look-out for a quick food fix.
- *Relevant chapter: Chapter 9, page 145. For good bedtime snack ideas, see the 'Pick the Right Snacks' section in the same chapter (page 159).*

Nicki's Tip

My favourite bedtime snack is a small bowl of porridge. I find it's satisfying without sitting heavily in my stomach (especially if I make it with half milk, half water). I add a sprinkling of sultanas or other dried fruit to give it a great natural sweetness.

Day 6: Get Your Body Moving
Why: If you're exercising, you're not only blowing away the cobwebs, you're also helping to change your brain chemistry.
If you suffer from sugar cravings and poor blood-sugar control, exercise will be a good friend to you. It helps your body deal with insulin better, balances blood-sugar and helps you gain muscle and lose fat.

Action

- **Find 'activity opportunities'.** When it comes to being fit and active, we're not saying you have to go down the gym. Every little bit of extra activity counts. For today, think about areas of your life where you could increase your level of activity. For example, do you always drive to the local shop even though it's two streets away? Do you cadge a lift to the station rather than leaving 10 minutes earlier to walk there instead? Organizations such as the British Heart Foundation are aware of how these extra steps each day can help us all as we strive for better health and fitness. Make today the day you start to incorporate more activity into your life.
- **Be active for 20 minutes a day.** This doesn't mean working out every day (three times a week is sufficient for that) but doing something that gets your heart rate rising a little, such as climbing stairs or walking.
- **Try Nicki's exercises.** Nicki devised the set of exercises in Chapter 10 to help her overcome her own sugar cravings.
- *Relevant chapter: Chapter 10, page 165.*

> ### Nicki's Tips
>
> *Becoming more active is a really important part of a healthy life. But as with anything, it's important not to overdo it. The reason? Over-exercising can put your adrenal glands under strain, increasing the levels of stress hormones in the blood and contributing to insulin resistance, which adds to problems with blood-sugar control.*
>
> *Just increase your activity levels a little by doing things you wouldn't normally do. Hide the remote control so you have to get up and switch channels; park the car down the road rather than outside your house so you have to walk to it. By getting yourself shifting, doing proper exercises won't feel like such a shock for your body!*

STAGE 3: KEEPING THE DIET UP
Days 7–13: Getting Used to Your New Food Routine
Why: This part of the plan is to help you make the new healthy-eating habits in Stage 2 your eating plan for life.

You'll go on to remove sugar from your diet, but whatever happens, this plan will give you the basics for a lifetime of healthy eating. The sugar removal is the 'icing on the cake' (so to speak!), the fine-tuning of this plan.

SUGAR ADDICTS' DIET

Eventually – as you'll see in Stage 5 – you'll get to the point where you'll be able to occasionally enjoy some foods from the 'Foods to avoid' list because your blood-sugar levels will be much more stable and your body should be better able to cope with them. But we've got some way to go before then. Keep up with the diet and you're one stage further towards that happening!

Action

- **Get familiar with Stage 2 of the plan**. From this point onwards, you should be strict with yourself about days 1–6. In other words, every day you should be having a proper breakfast, eating three meals, 'smart' snacking, discovering new drinks, eating before bed and getting your body moving. The idea is that at the end of these 13 days, you should be starting to feel like your blood-sugar is beginning to stabilize and your sugar highs and lows are evening out.
- **See it as a way of getting 'back on track'**. Whatever happens, you can always use these first seven days as the basis for getting things back on track. If, for example, when you've been advised to cut down on sugar later on, you find yourself straying and splurging on all your old favourites, start back on track by implementing days 1–6.
- **Move on when you feel comfortable**. Ideally, you should be moving on to day 14 as soon as you've finished days 7–13. But the next stage of the diet is all

The 21-day Plan

about giving up that added sugar, and you may find it's the most difficult stage. There's no point in us telling you to move on to this stage if you don't feel ready – you might find you don't stick to it. Perhaps you've got too much going on in your life at the moment and it doesn't seem like the right time to make such a momentous step. The answer? Stick to days 7–13 (Stage 3 of the diet) until you feel ready to move on.

- **Keep writing your diary**. Also, don't forget to keep referring back to your goals to help you focus on why you're doing this.
- *Relevant chapters: Chapters 8 (page 119), 9 (page 145), 10 (page 165) and 14 (page 285).*

Nicki's Tip

Don't punish yourself if you've slipped. If, for example, you've found yourself unable to stick with brown carbohydrates for every meal and snack, don't just give up. Ideally, you should be eating brown but the most important thing at this stage is that you combine protein and carbohydrate, as this'll help balance your blood-sugar levels. If you're not feeling all over the place, you're more likely to make rational decisions about food choices.

SUGAR ADDICTS' DIET

STAGE 4: QUITTING SUGAR
Day 14: Be a Sugar 'Detective'

Why: This is to help you see where sugars are 'hiding' and take note of foods that are likely to trip you up as you try to reduce sugar in your diet.

This is technically your first day of really starting to think about cutting down on sugar. Don't be daunted – you've already partly done it. Remember reading about refined carbohydrates in Chapter 3? There we told you about how they act like pure sugars in your body. So if you've managed to make some changes from white to brown products, you've already cut some sugar out of your diet. This next stage is to empower you to 'detect' some of those other places where sugars are found.

Action

- **Get to know your sugars**. As you discovered in Chapter 8, sugar doesn't always come under the name 'sugar'. Read the section 'Recognizing Sugars' on pages 130–31 again to familiarize yourself with some of the 'other' names for sugar. You'll see from the list that sugar comes in many disguises. But if you get used to reading labels, you'll soon find 'sugar-spotting' becomes second-nature.
- **Spend time 'spotting' sugars**. Read labels of foods you have in your home to prove to yourself just how commonplace they are. If you pop out to a sandwich bar at lunchtime or to the local shop or supermarket,

The 21-day Plan

do the same thing. By law, products must have their ingredients listed so you should find them on all packaged foods you pick up.

- **Use sticky labels**. Get some plain sticky labels in a bright colour such as red. Put a label on each food you find in your cupboards or fridge which contains added sugar or is in the 'Refined/sneaky sugars' list in Chapter 8. When you see lots of red-labelled foods next to each other, you'll begin to understand just how many of them – or how few of them – there are in your life. You could buy another colour – say, green – for your non-sugar or complex foods. As the weeks go by, you should be stocking more green foods than red. This will help you to 'audit' your food cupboards to know whether you're on the right track or still harbouring those sugars you love so much!
- **Some label advice**. On a food label the ingredients are listed from those that are present in the greatest quantity to those in the smallest quantity. So if an ingredients list says 'Water, salt, oranges, sugar', it has more water in it than oranges. If it says 'Sugar, oranges, salt, water', it has more sugar in it than water.
- **Identify your sugar 'threats'**. Work out where the biggest threats to you being sugar-free actually come from and get some strategies in place (see Chapter 12).
- ***Relevant chapters:** Chapter 8 (page 119), Chapter 12 (page 201).*

> **Nicki's Tip**
>
> *Carry out your own mini 'survey' when you next go shopping. Choose 10 pre-prepared foods such as tins or packets that you'd normally buy. For example, look at the labels of ketchup, pasta sauces and ice cream that are on your usual shopping list. See how many out of that 10 contain sugar. I often end up doing more than 10 – 'sugar spotting' is addictive!*

Day 15: Clear Out Your Kitchen

Why: Now you've spotted where the sugars are, it's time to get rid of the foods containing obvious sugars.

Action

- **Isolate your sugary foods.** We don't mean put them at the end of the garden (though that might work for some people!). You've got to be realistic – if you have a family that loves sugary food then you might have mutiny on your hands if you try and bin the lot. But it's not going to do you any favours if it's sitting there tempting you. If you have to have it around, come up with a strategy. Put the sweet things in a cupboard you don't normally go to so those sweet foods won't 'wink' at you every time you open the door.

- **Make healthy foods 'convenience foods'.** You know how it is – if that chocolate's there, you'll eat it. Believe it or not, the same will happen with healthy foods if you start to put them in places where you'd normally get your sugar 'kick'. Make things convenient to encourage you to eat them – chop up a batch of vegetables such as carrot, baby sweetcorn and cucumber to munch on and keep them in a plastic box in the fridge, or keep a sandwich bag with some mixed nuts in your coat pocket or handbag to give you access to a quick snack when you're out.
- **Work with your own habits.** If you know you're a creature of habit then work with those habits instead of fighting against them. If they're the right habits, they can be a boost to healthy living so turn them around. For example, if you know you always have a 'high' at 6pm because you eat chocolate, replace that 'high' with a walk with the dog, a phone call to a friend or even a romantic moment with your partner.
- **Try out new gadgets.** If you haven't already tried out any new gadgets you've bought to help you kick sugar, now's the time. Whether it's a popcorn maker, a blender or ice-lolly makers, try them out. The more familiar you get with them, the more confidence you'll have in using them for all kinds of sugar-free options. See Chapter 11, page 197.
- ***Relevant chapter:** Chapter 11, page 191.*

Day 16: Preparing Your Sugar Alternatives

Why: This is to help you get the right snacks and sugar alternatives in place so you know what you can eat and what you should avoid on day 18, the 'big day'.

This is important – human nature means as soon as someone says you can't have something, you want it! If you have good alternatives in place, you shouldn't find yourself so tempted to reach for chocolate, sweets or cakes.

Action

- **Think 'variety'.** If you have only one alternative in place, you're soon going to feel like you're being punished. The key here is to have many different sweet alternatives to hand. Try frozen fruit, fruit and nut mixtures, smoothies, yoghurt with muesli, shop-bought bars and fruit-sweetened popcorn. There are endless possibilities to ensure you don't get bored of the same taste.
- **Discover new fruits.** Fruit isn't just apples and oranges. Supermarkets stock all kinds of interesting fruit that you might not even have tried before. These fruits can be eaten alone or used to sweeten foods. For example, mango is a wonderful, naturally sweet fruit that is great when mixed with yoghurt, like a thick shake. Some of these 'exotic' fruits may look a bit odd to you, but don't be put off.

- **Get your friends and family ready.** You'll have picked up some great tips on how to deal with all the people and situations in your life that seem to drive you towards sugar. But with a couple of days to go, it's worth letting people know that you're soon going to be giving up sugar. Ask friends, family and colleagues to be supportive and not tempt you with sweets or other foods you're trying to avoid. Most people will probably be a little curious but supportive. If they're teasing you, think back to your 'goals' list on day 1 of your diary, and, as you turn down their offer of chocolate cake, tell them, 'You might think it's strange but maybe you won't when I'm thinner/healthier/less spotty.'
- *Relevant chapters: Chapter 11, page 191, Chapter 15, page 295.*

Nicki's Tip

If you're after flavours you normally associate with sweet foods but don't want the sugar, try adding pure vanilla essence or cinnamon to food or drinks.

Day 17: Learning to Say 'No'

Why: At this point, you're likely to be 'drawn in' by people or situations encouraging you to eat sugar. Here are some tips on learning to say 'no' to your 'dealers'.

Action

- **Learn to say 'no' to your dealers.** The 'dealers' in our lives vary from person to person but there are some key situations that affect most of us. See Chapter 12 for coping strategies.
- **Spot your own dealers**. Take a look at Chapter 12 and put a mark next to the sections that relate most to your life. Go through and find the strategy or strategies you think will most help you to cope.

Day 18: The Big Day

Why: Your first sugar-free day! You're going to be saying 'no' to your normal sugary or 'white' favourites (such as cakes and biscuits).

This day had to come at some point, but more than two weeks after starting the diet, you have plenty of tools to make this great leap forward. Under normal circumstances, detoxing generally takes five days, and going 'cold turkey' could leave you feeling grumpy, headachy and desperate for a sugar fix. But the aim of the plan up to this point has been to help stabilize your blood-sugar levels and give you a good, healthy, balanced diet so that your body can cope easily with the 'blow' of not having its sugar fix.

Action
- **Set the scene for giving up sugar.** Make sure you choose a good time to do it – for example, if you get to day 17 and it's the worst possible day because it's in the middle of a house move or the kids' exams, don't force yourself to stop eating sugar today. If you're stressed, you're more likely to reach for a 'pick-me-up'. And if you're reading this book, chances are that boost will be a sweet food! Of course, you can start on a stressful day if you want to but leave it until another day if it feels like it's going to put you under extra strain. If this is the case, keep going with days 1–8 and choose your first sugar-free day when things calm down.
- **Get some good distractions in place.** You can't have a chocolate bar or custard cream so it's guaranteed that's what you want the most! When you're giving something up – whether it's sugar or nicotine – it's best to have something to occupy your hands and your head to stop you focusing on what you can't have. Good examples include crosswords, playing cards, sewing, knitting, painting or even DIY. If you don't do any of these, now's the time to start!
- **Understand you might not feel 100 per cent.** Although we hope you won't be feeling ratty, low or

headachy, it may happen to you. Or you may feel edgy knowing you can't have sugar. But chances are it'll be psychological because, if you've stuck to the diet, your blood-sugar should have stabilized and your cravings subsided. If you feel this way, don't worry – you're not alone and it's not a sign that you should eat sugar again to feel better. If you're feeling really bad, look at day 19 for some tips on how to cope.

- **Get some support**. Have friends on standby to call or visit on this potentially difficult day. They don't have to be doing the diet, too – all you need is someone you can talk it through with. If you're visiting them, ask them not to offer you sweet foods or to eat them in front of you. Take your own snacks with you so you're not tempted.
- **Remember your goals**. On day 1 you wrote a list of goals to help you stay focused in your bid to give up sugar. If you haven't been looking at these goals each day, now is the day to take a really good look at them and to concentrate on all the reasons why quitting sugar will benefit you.

> **Nicki's Tip**
>
> *Accept that you may well feel terrible. This really is a classic example of 'no pain, no gain'. I had terrible headaches when I tried to quit sugar without supporting my body through it with a healthy diet. Learn from my experience and get your diet under control before you quit. By doing everything the plan suggests – including combining carbs with protein and finding good sugar substitutes – your side-effects won't be half as bad as they would have been. You shouldn't feel like this for long.*

Day 19: Lifting Your Mood without Sugar

Why: You're likely to feel pretty crummy today. Your body could well be telling you, 'Eat sugar, eat sugar!' and you might have a tough time resisting it. But here are some hints and tips on how to handle this potentially difficult day – and make the next few easier, too.

Action

- **Replacing that feeling.** Many of us reach for sugar when we're feeling physically 'yuk' or emotional in some way (such as when we're sad or even happy). It gives us a physical or emotional lift (or both). Write a list of activities you enjoy (such as watching comedy on television, listening to a CD, painting a picture) plus things you've been meaning to do for ages (ring a friend, weed the garden). Make it a nice long list and put all kinds of things on it, from those that are easy to accomplish through to big projects. When you get a sugar craving, select an item from the list to carry out. Not only will this help distract you from your sweet craving, it's also likely to give you a different 'high' (such as from laughing at a joke or some good, hard physical labour in the garden). Keep adding to the list – and always make the additions positive ones for good motivation.

- **Rely on your sugar 'alternatives'.** We're not saying you should eat these until they come out of your ears (if the plan works for you then you shouldn't want to eat that many anyway), but remember they're there to help you overcome your need for added sugar. Use them!

- **Think 'convenience'.** No, we don't mean ready meals or fast foods, but there's a lot to be said for having your healthy meals and snacks at the ready. This avoids situations where you have to eat now and the only thing available is a cake. If you know you're likely to stray, make sure your snacks are to hand (for example, always have healthy snacks in your desk so you're not tempted by the vending machine or tea trolley) and your meals aren't so elaborate and

ambitious that they take for ever to cook and you eat biscuits while you're waiting.
- **Exercise**. If you haven't done Nicki's exercises yet, now's the time to really get into them. The 'feel-good' endorphins released by exercise will help to give you a high you might otherwise have sought from sugary foods (see Chapter 10).

Nicki's Tip

Give yourself a treat a day. And I don't mean a food treat. But it's got to be something that makes you feel good about yourself. On the first day of giving up sugar, write a list of treats that you're going to give yourself over the next few days – at least one for each day.

Day 20: Give Yourself a Supplement Boost
Why: In an ideal world, if you have a good diet, you shouldn't need supplements. But even with a well-balanced diet there are a number of reasons why supplements may be helpful.

Firstly, food isn't as nutritious as it used to be – refining and processing deplete nutrients as do cooking styles, low levels of soil nutrients, modern living and pollution. Secondly, higher doses of vitamins and minerals than the RDA (recommended daily amounts) may help you safely support your body as you try to regulate blood-sugar levels and quash your cravings.

Certain nutrients are said to help with cravings (see below). Experts say that a good multivitamin containing all of these should help provide you with the nutrients you need, boosting the levels you're getting through healthy eating. If you want an extra 'boost', you could try a product like SucroGuard by BioCare which has been devised specifically to control levels of glucose in the blood. You may decide that taking supplements is something you don't want to do – that's fine, and of course it's entirely your choice. Nicki found it helped her but you may be happiest trying to stick with food alone. There's no right or wrong here!

Remember – if you're going to take supplements, you should understand that vitamins and minerals depend on each other to work properly. Rather than taking individual ones in isolation, a multivitamin is a good baseline and 'insurance policy'. For further information about dietary supplements, it's worth consulting a nutritional therapist (visit the British Association of Nutritional Therapists www.bant.org.uk for further information and to find your nearest therapist).

Women who are pregnant or thinking of having a baby are advised by the Food Standards Agency to avoid taking supplements containing vitamin A. Although it isn't in SucroGuard, vitamin A is usually found in multivitamins. However, you can buy multivitamins specially formulated for conception and pregnancy which don't contain vitamin A. Speak to your GP or nutritionist if you need further advice.

Multivitamin Supplements
- Go for a multivitamin containing vitamin C, vitamin B complex (a selection of B vitamins, especially B_1, B_2, B_3 and B_6), chromium, magnesium, manganese and zinc. SucroGuard contains all of these but in slightly higher levels than a multivitamin so it may be worth taking in addition to your multivitamin for an extra boost.

Minerals
- **Chromium**. This helps balance blood-sugar levels and control insulin. If you are sedentary, your insulin levels will be higher and therefore your need for chromium will be greater. Lack of activity also leads to chromium being depleted, so being sedentary could be helping to fuel your cravings. A moderate amount of exercise helps your body retain chromium (see Chapter 10 for advice on how to get more active). Good foods for chromium include Marmite, prunes, wheat germ, raw mushrooms and rye bread. A diet high in sugar and refined carbohydrates can deplete your chromium intake by up to 97 per cent. You may find that extra chromium helps you to ditch added sugar in your diet.

- **Magnesium**. This helps support insulin function so is vital for blood-sugar levels. It is also involved in the production of the 'feel-good' chemical serotonin, as well as being vital for energy. Low levels of magnesium can make you feel low, stressed or lacking in energy. All of these might then have you reaching for sweet foods to make you feel happier or more energized. Good foods for magnesium include wheat germ, almonds, Marmite, Brazil nuts and hazelnuts.
- **Manganese**. This is an important part of blood-sugar control and essential for the breakdown of carbohydrates and proteins. Good food sources include beetroot, blackberries, oats and raspberries.
- **Zinc**. Vital for insulin function as it is involved in its production and in helping cells to be more reactive to insulin. Studies have shown that low zinc levels are associated with increased levels of insulin resistance and even diabetes. Zinc is also an important mineral for the production of serotonin and is needed for proper food digestion (it's essential for the production of stomach acid). Good food sources include oysters, wheat germ, sesame seeds, pumpkin seeds and turkey.

Vitamins
- **B vitamins**. These all work together, but if you're craving carbohydrates such as sugar the key ones you may be deficient in are B_3, B_6 and biotin. The B vitamins are also important for energy production so

you may be feeling washed out if you're lacking in them. B_3 works with chromium to help balance blood-sugar levels, B_6 helps to balance hormones (including insulin) while biotin is needed to turn carbohydrates into glucose and to control blood-sugar levels (it can help to lower raised blood-sugar). B_5 is also vital to support your adrenal glands, which are important for blood-sugar levels. In fact, low levels can contribute to low blood sugar. Good food sources of B_3 include wholegrain cereals, chicken and oily fish (such as tuna and salmon). B_6 is found in wholegrain cereals, sunflower seeds, muesli and sesame seeds. Biotin is contained in walnuts, almonds, eggs and peas. Foods containing B_5 include mushrooms, oatmeal and soy beans.

- **Vitamin C**. This is needed to produce the stress hormones adrenaline and cortisol in your adrenal glands. Low blood-sugar levels and adrenal exhaustion (when your adrenal glands are overworked, such as during stress) are closely linked so it's vital to keep vitamin C levels up to normalize blood-sugar. Fruit and vegetables are rich sources of vitamin C.

Day 21: Keeping Your Motivation Up

At this stage you're likely to be wondering, 'What difference is this going to make to my life?' You may have had positive experiences on the diet so far, as Nicki did very early on. She also lost five pounds in two weeks.

However, it may be that you're still fighting your sugar urges and missing your sweet foods (despite our suggestions for alternatives). If you're one of these people, Nicki has a message for you:

'*Please* stick with it! This isn't a faddy diet. It's a healthy eating plan. Not only will it help stabilize your blood-sugar levels to get your sugar cravings under control, it'll also do wonders for your body and health. When I first saw the plan, I wasn't convinced I'd ever get to the stage where I wouldn't be craving sugar as much as I did. But I stuck with it, going through every day of the plan in the hope it would make a difference. Within days I started to feel much more "on a level", and by day 21 I was feeling like a new woman. I had more energy than I could ever have hoped for, I needed less sleep and the bags under my eyes had gone. People were commenting on my rosy cheeks and fantastic complexion. But, most importantly, my cravings had subsided and my body fat had definitely gone down. Even at this early stage, the pounds were dropping off me.'

Here are Nicki's suggestions for keeping your motivation up:

- **Give yourself goals worth striving for**. Any goal has to be something you really want, or it's no goal at all. It could be that outfit you've hung in the bedroom as a reminder of how much weight you'd like to shed. Or it could be that page you've torn out of the holiday

brochure to remind yourself of that dream destination you'll go to when you look better in a swimming costume. And keep creating these goals – there's no reason why you should have only one (short-term goals are vital for motivation, too).
- **Remember how sugar makes you feel**. If you've been sticking to the diet, it may be that it's a while since you've had any sugar, and you may have forgotten how it makes you feel. Keep sight of why you're trying to cut back. Make a list like this: Weight-loss, improved concentration, better skin, less prone to illness, not so moody. If you need help compiling it, turn back to your diary and write down some of the negative words. Keep a copy of the list in your purse to stop you when you're about to buy chocolate, or in the family biscuit tin.
- **Imagine sugar making you fat**. Think of all the places where that kilo of pick 'n' mix could go if you scoff it all – visualize your 'trouble spots' such as your thighs or bum, and imagine it going straight there and creating a big 'wobble'. Or see it heading towards your brain to give you a headache. Sounds extreme but if it stops you eating it, let your imagination run wild!
- **That's what friends are for**. And families, for that matter. Both friends and relatives are likely to be a vital part of your success when it comes to sticking to the Sugar Addicts' Diet. They can be 'dealers' but they

can also help you achieve your goals. Help them to keep you motivated – offer to give them lists of the foods you are and aren't allowed so they can help you steer clear of them.
- **Have a sweet experience ... without the sweets**. Treating yourself doesn't have to be with food. When you're tempted to eat something sweet, do something else you enjoy instead. It could be having a long bath, listening to some favourite music, ringing a friend, reading a magazine or novel or watching a video or programmes you've recorded and haven't had time to watch. Make a list of these sweet experiences so you can treat yourself to one next time you're heading for the sugar.

STAGE 5: WHAT NEXT?

You might be wondering whether this now means a life without sugary foods. The point of the diet – as well as helping you cut out sugar to lose weight – is to get your blood-sugar stable. This helps minimize cravings so that you won't feel the need to have so much added sugar. But we know that once in a while you'll really want it – and as far as we're concerned there's no reason why you shouldn't have an occasional sugary treat. But the aim here is to get you on to the Sugar Addicts' Diet and make it your new eating plan before you start to allow yourself these treats. Once you're eating properly, you should find – as Nicki has – that you can eat sweet foods

The 21-day Plan

occasionally without your blood-sugar levels going all over the place.

In a nutshell, make this plan your new way of life, and within weeks you should no longer have such dire cravings. You'll also be able to eat occasional sugary treats without going back to your old ways.

14
Menu Plans

GETTING THE BALANCE RIGHT

This 21-day plan gives you a daily intake of five carbohydrate portions, two to three protein portions, two to three dairy portions and at least five portions of fruit and veg (see Chapter 8, page 119). It also allows for your healthy snacks (see Chapter 9, page 159).

Some days you may have more of one food group, but it balances out over the course of the week. We've planned these menus to give you a healthy mix of foods that add up to a daily calorific value of 1,500–2,000 – perfect for a good steady weight loss in combination with regular exercise, such as Nicki's routine (see Chapter 10).

At the end of this chapter there is advice on using the plan, and some tips from Nicki on making it easy to follow.

WEEK 1	MONDAY	TUESDAY	WEDNESDAY	THURSDAY	FRIDAY	SATURDAY	SUNDAY
BREAKFAST	3 tbsp unsweetened muesli with 200ml skimmed milk	1–2 slices of Vogel or Burgen bread toasted with 2 tsp of peanut butter and a glass of orange juice	Smoothie – e.g. Mixed Berry Smoothie (p. 297)	Cinnamon Sultana Toast (p. 297) (2 slices) and a glass of orange juice	1–2 slices of Vogel or Burgen bread toasted with 2 tsp of peanut butter and a glass of orange juice	Porridge (4–5 tbsp), sultanas, nuts and 1 tsp plain yoghurt	2 slices of granary toast with scrambled egg (2 eggs, a little low-fat milk and 1 tsp of olive spread) and smoked salmon (1 slice flaked) plus a slice of melon
LUNCH	2 wholemeal pitta pockets with 2 tbsp of reduced-fat houmous with grated carrot, chopped red pepper, lettuce and tomato and a glass of orange juice	2 slices of granary bread with egg 'mayo' (1 hardboiled egg mixed with 1 egg, 2 tbsp 'mayo' and chives) with tomato. Plus 1 portion of fruit (e.g. an apple)	2 slices of rye bread with 3 thin slices of ham and 1 tsp of Dijon mustard served with a side salad of rocket, cherry tomatoes, spring onion and a balsamic vinegar dressing. Plus 1 portion of fruit (e.g. a pear)	2 slices of granary toast (or multigrain bread) with 2 tbsp tuna or sardine pâté. Plus 1 portion of fruit (e.g. a small bunch of grapes)	Jacket potato with 1 tsp of low-fat cream cheese (instead of butter) and a small can of sugar-free baked beans (with a dash of soy or Worcester sauce). 100g pot of plain yoghurt plus chopped fruit or fruit mix	Feta, Olive and Baby New Potato Salad (p. 314) (with plenty of salad vegetables). Plus 1 portion of fruit (e.g. 3 plums)	Serving of New Covent Garden pumpkin soup (or any fresh – rather than tinned – soup) with a multigrain roll. 100g pot of plain yoghurt with 1 portion of fruit (e.g. an apple)

DINNER	'Meaty' Bolognaise (p. 308) with spaghetti plus 1 bowl of mixed salad	Chicken and Cashew Stir-fry (p. 306) with egg noodles	Chilli Bean Wraps (p. 301)	Fettuccini Carbonara (p. 311) with a bowl of mixed salad	Fresh grilled tuna, sweet potato wedges plus a side salad	Curry of choice (see 'Quick' Curry, p. 305) with 3 tbsp basmati rice	Roast of choice. Avoid: mashed potato, mashed swede, fatty meat Choose: baby new potatoes (boiled and/or roasted), plus plenty of fresh veg, e.g. cauliflower. Lean meat (see below)

WEEK 2	MONDAY	TUESDAY	WEDNESDAY	THURSDAY	FRIDAY	SATURDAY	SUNDAY
BREAKFAST	Smoothie of choice (e.g. Mixed Berry, p. 297)	Porridge (4–5 tbsp), sultanas, nuts and 1 tsp plain yoghurt	Smoothie of choice (e.g. Pear and Peach, p. 297)	Porridge (4–5 tbsp), sultanas, nuts and 1 tsp plain yoghurt	2 slices of Vogel or Burgen bread toasted with 1 tbsp of low-fat cream cheese and Marmite and a glass of apple or orange juice	Cinnamon Sultana Toast (p.297) (2 slices) and a glass of orange juice	2 rashers of lean grilled bacon, a poached egg and a grilled tomato with 2 tbsp sugar-free baked beans
LUNCH	45g mozzarella cheese with sliced tomato and basil in a wrap with a glass of apple or pineapple juice	2 slices of granary bread with 1 tbsp prawn 'mayo' with lettuce. 100g pot of low-fat yoghurt and 1 portion of fruit (e.g a small bunch of grapes)	Jacket potato with tuna and sweetcorn 'mayo' (small can of tuna in spring water, 1 tbsp of sweetcorn – from sugar-free can – and 1 tbsp 'mayo'). Plus 1 portion of fruit (e.g. an apple)	Grilled chicken and pasta salad with a glass of pineapple juice. 100g pot of plain yoghurt plus 1 portion of fruit (e.g. fruit mix)	Fresh lentil soup (e.g. New Covent Garden or other fresh variety, not tinned) with a granary or multigrain roll. 100g pot of plain yoghurt with 1 portion of fruit (e.g a small punnet of raspberries)	Grilled Edam (45g) with tomato and Worcester sauce on 2 slices of granary toast and a small can of pineapple in juice	Roast of choice. Avoid: mashed potato, mashed swede, fatty meat. Choose: baby new potatoes (boiled and/or roasted), plus plenty of fresh veg. Lean meat (see below)

| DINNER | Beef and Lentil Burgers (p. 312) with a mixed salad | Grilled chicken breast with corn on the cob and Carrot and Sultana Salad (p. 321) | Tuna Macaroni Bake (p. 326) with green vegetables (broccoli, spinach or French beans) | Sweet Potato and Leek Frittata (p.313) with a mixed green salad | Grilled salmon steak with 4–5 baby new potatoes and broccoli, mangetout and carrots | Home-made curry of choice (e.g. chicken) with 3 tbsp basmati rice | Omelette of choice (p. 299) and a bowl of salad plus 2 rye crispbreads with light spread (don't have crispbreads if omelette is Spanish, i.e. with potatoes) |

WEEK 3	MONDAY	TUESDAY	WEDNESDAY	THURSDAY	FRIDAY	SATURDAY	SUNDAY
BREAKFAST	Smoothie of choice (e.g. 'Chocolate' Banana smoothie, p. 297)	1–2 slices of Vogel or Burgen bread toasted with 2 tsp of peanut butter and a glass of skimmed milk	Smoothie of choice (e.g. Mango and Strawberry, p. 297)	2 slices of Vogel or Burgen bread toasted with 1 tbsp of low-fat cream cheese and Marmite. Plus a glass of apple or orange juice	Porridge (4–5 tbsp), sultanas, nuts and 1 tsp plain yoghurt	Cinnamon Sultana Toast (p. 297) and a glass of orange juice	Omelette of choice (e.g. 'Meaty', p. 299), slice of grainy toast plus a glass of juice
LUNCH	2 slices of granary bread with very low-fat spread, 3 thin slices of turkey ham, sliced tomato, a pear and 1 slice of Edam	2 slices of Vogel or Burgen bread with 45g Brie and sliced grapes on top. Plus 1 portion of fruit (e.g. an apple)	2 slices of pumpernickel bread with very low-fat spread, topped with 2 slices of smoked salmon, sliced cucumber and dill. Plus 1 portion of fruit (e.g. 1 small bunch of grapes)	Sweet Pasta Salad (p. 322) with tuna (100g). 100g pot of low-fat yoghurt plus 1 portion of fruit (e.g. small punnet of strawberries)	2 pitta pockets with 4 falafel (see below), chilli sauce and shredded lettuce and 100g pot of low-fat yoghurt	Mexican Quorn Wrap (p. 303) plus 1 portion of fruit (e.g. 4 fresh apricots)	Roast of choice. Avoid: mashed potato, mashed swede, fatty meat. Choose: baby new potatoes (boiled and/or roasted), plus plenty of fresh veg. Lean meat (see below)

DINNER	Quorn Lasagne (p. 309) with sweetcorn and mangetout	Prawn stir-fry with egg noodles	Spanish omelette (p. 300) and bowl of mixed salad	Sausage and Apple Casserole (p. 315) with 3 small jacket potatoes	Herby Cod Fillets (p. 316) with 3 small baked potatoes and ratatouille	Curry of choice (e.g. Creamy Vegetable Curry, p. 305) and 3 tbsp basmati rice	Rye crispbread and/or granary toast with cheese (e.g. Edam, Philadelphia Light, Brie, low-fat mozzarella, cottage cheese). Plus 1 portion of fruit (e.g. apple)

ADVICE ON THE PLAN

- **Roast dinner of choice.** Each Sunday we're giving you the chance to have a roast dinner. Whether you have it for lunch or in the evening is up to you. The rest of the day's food has been made 'light' on purpose to accommodate this weekly treat. A roast dinner can be balanced and healthy if you eat it right. Choose lean meat such as chicken or turkey, or a chop. Always bake or roast rather than frying. Always remove the skin, rind or any visible fat. Avoid mashed potatoes and swede, which have a high GI and opt instead for a small portion of tiny new potatoes. These are great when boiled and can also be roasted in a little olive oil as a weekly treat. Get your portions right – use the list in Chapter 9 to ensure you don't have too much of anything. But remember – when it comes to healthy veg, you can have as much as you like, so fill up on that.
- **Daily milk allowance.** Each day you're allowed 300ml of skimmed or semi-skimmed milk for use in drinks (e.g. coffee substitutes) or to drink on its own. If it's a day when you have a smoothie, remember that 100ml of that allowance will be used to make this recipe up. You should also count any milk used on cereal.
- **Falafel.** These are spicy balls made with ground chickpeas, popular in the Middle East. Most supermarkets stock a falafel mix so you can make up your own, or you can buy it ready-made.

Menu Plans

- **Desserts**. Traditional sweet desserts are not included in the plan because they are meant to be occasional treats. You can allow yourself one portion of dessert a week – perhaps at the weekend – but only if you want it. However, on several days of the plan we have included yoghurt and fruit options.
- **Breakfast**. In Chapter 9 we gave you a list of cereals you can eat (page 155). For variety, you can incorporate these into the 21-day plan, if you like.

Nicki's Tips

Cook in bulk. Make up a batch of Bolognaise mix and freeze it in portion sizes to suit your lifestyle, such as single portions for one person or family-sized portions. Also, make up a batch of fruit mix and keep it in the fridge for a couple of days. Alternatively, freeze it in an ice-cube tray and transfer to a freezer bag, then take out as many cubes as you need and allow them to defrost before use.

Buy frozen herbs. If you want the taste of fresh herbs but can never find them (or always kill them when you try to grow them!) buy them frozen. Look in the freezer section of your supermarket to find small, easy-to-store boxes of herbs and ready chopped garlic.

Freeze your loaf. A 'grainy' loaf may be more expensive than the bread you'd normally buy. If it's only you eating it and not your family, keep the loaf in the freezer so you can bring out each slice when you need it. That way you can make sure it doesn't go mouldy before you've had a chance to eat it! Also, if it's there, you won't be tempted to stray to the white loaf your family's eating if yours runs out…

Mix up nuts and seeds. Buy a bag of mixed nuts, put them in a screw-top jar (like an old jam or pasta sauce jar) or a large sandwich bag. Add some seeds, such as pumpkin seeds, sunflower seeds and sesame seeds. That way, when you want a handful of nuts and seeds, you just shake up the bag or jar (the smallest ones always settle at the bottom) and grab some.

Undercook pasta. Yes, really! Pasta that is 'al dente' (in other words, slightly undercooked) has a lower GI than if you cook it so it's sloppy. As well as having a better texture (after all, that's how the Italians eat it) it'll be a better form of slow-release energy.

15

Recipes to Help You Give Up Sugar

BREAKFASTS

Smoothies

These are fantastic shakes that anyone can enjoy, particularly those who can't stomach breakfast! They contain protein and good refined carbohydrates (from the crispbread and fruit) to give you plenty of energy. Smoothies also make great snacks at any time of the day.

We've given you various flavour options to use in combination with the basic smoothie recipe. But experiment – we're finding different flavour combinations all the time.

If you don't have a liquidizer, it might be time to invest in one. It will save you having to chop your fruit and nuts into small pieces by hand. You can buy a liquidizer or hand blender for under £20.

SUGAR ADDICTS' DIET

Basic Smoothie Recipe

Serves 1
- 2 rye crispbreads (e.g. Ryvita)
- 3 tbsp plain live yoghurt
- 100ml low-fat milk
- Vanilla essence

Strawberry Shortcake Flavourings
- 6 dried apricots
- 100g strawberries (about 6–8 medium strawberries)
- Handful of whole almonds (about 6–8)

Crush the crispbread in a liquidizer, or put into a sandwich bag and crush with a rolling pin or can of beans). Add the rest of the ingredients and liquidize or whisk until smooth. Pour half the mixture into a glass and serve chilled.

Variations
- Take the Basic Smoothie Recipe and add extra ingredients to make the following:

Mango and Strawberry Smoothie
Really sweet and delicious! Add 100g mango and 100g strawberries.

Recipes to Help You Give Up Sugar

Mixed Berry Smoothie
Add 100g strawberries, 50g raspberries and 50g blueberries plus 6 dried apricots to sweeten.

Pear and Peach Smoothie
Add 1 piece of each fruit plus 6 dried apricots. If you don't have fresh fruit, use tinned pears (100g without the liquid) and peaches in their own juice (not syrup). Note: tinned fruit tends to make a runnier smoothie.

'Chocolate' Banana Smoothie
Add 1 banana (the softer the banana, the sweeter the taste!) plus 1 tsp of carob powder for a 'chocolate-style' smoothie.

Cinnamon Sultana Toast

We love this. If you like the taste of hot cross buns, you'll love it, too. This makes a great snack as well as a breakfast food.

Serves 2
- 1 tsp ground cinnamon
- 50g sultanas or raisins
- 4 tsp low-fat cream cheese (e.g. Philadelphia Light) or quark
- 4 slices granary bread
- Mix the cinnamon and dried fruit with the cream cheese. Spread on toast and enjoy! It's that easy!

Variation
- Make a very low-fat version using cottage cheese.

Fruit Mix

This is great to eat at breakfast with unsweetened muesli, porridge or yoghurt, but you can also have it with custard and pancakes as a dessert.

Serves 2
  1 apple, diced
  1 pear (or small tin of pears)
  1 peach (or small tin of peaches)
  ½ tsp ground cinnamon
  4 prunes (or 2 tbsp sultanas)
  1 tbsp mixed nuts
  1 glass of fresh orange juice

Put all the ingredients except the orange juice in a saucepan and cook gently for about 30 minutes, until the mixture thickens. If you're using tinned fruit, add up to 100ml of the juice to prevent the fruit from sticking to the pan. If using fresh fruit, add about 100ml of water, as required. Add the orange juice and cook until the mixture thickens again. Liquidize until it forms a paste. Chill for 2–3 hours then serve with yoghurt, muesli, porridge or custard.

Variations
- Use vanilla or almonds instead of cinnamon.
- Choose any fruits or unsweetened fruit juice you fancy.

Omelettes

You can add whatever you like to this standard omelette recipe, depending on how you feel and what's in the cupboard. To make one omelette, simply use half the ingredients listed below.

Makes 2
   4 eggs
   1 tbsp cold water
   Knob of butter
   Black pepper to taste

Put the eggs and water in a bowl and beat with a fork. Melt the butter in a frying pan, making sure the bottom and sides are coated with butter. When it bubbles, put the mixture in. Wiggle the pan so that the mixture runs from the middle to the sides, helping it to cook. Cook until the top of the omelette is creamy and the bottom has set. Fold one side over the other and serve.

Variations
Spanish Omelette
To turn the omelette into a Spanish omelette, you will need:

- 1 small onion, chopped
- ½ red pepper, chopped
- ½ green pepper, chopped
- 100g new potatoes including their skins, sliced

Before adding the egg mixture, put the onions, peppers and potatoes into the frying pan and cook until the potatoes are lightly browned. Then add the egg mixture and continue as for the basic omelette recipe.

Mushroom Omelette
Add 50g of sliced mushrooms (whatever variety you like) plus some fresh parsley to the mixture as it cooks.

'Meaty' Omelette
Add diced Quorn sausages to the mixture or 2 slices of turkey or chicken, cut into strips, plus 1 tomato, diced.

Other foods that work well in omelettes include smoked salmon, mozzarella cheese, Edam cheese.

Recipes to Help You Give Up Sugar

LUNCH/DINNER

Wraps

Saying you don't have time to cook is no excuse when these delicious wraps can be rustled up in the time it takes to microwave a ready-meal. Anyone who says healthy food is boring should try these – the red, yellow, green and purple from the vegetables makes them look fantastic and taste even better.

Chilli Bean Wraps

Serves 4
If you're making this for two people, you can freeze or chill the extra chilli sauce and have it the next day with a jacket potato or with some tortilla chips as a snack. If you're not sure about kidney beans, you can mash them up or liquidize them before putting them in the mixture.

Chilli Bean Sauce
- 1 medium red onion, chopped
- ½ red pepper, chopped
- 1 tbsp olive oil
- 200g Quorn mince (or chicken or turkey mince)
- 3 tbsp water
- 1 tsp soy sauce

SUGAR ADDICTS' DIET

- ½ tsp chilli powder or Tabasco sauce
- 1 can red kidney beans (400g)
- 1 can tomatoes (400g)
- 8 corn tortillas or 12 taco shells
- 2 tbsp low-fat cream cheese
- 60g Edam cheese, grated

Cook the onion and pepper in a frying pan with the olive oil until the onions are turning transparent. Add the mince and cook until golden brown, adding a little water to stop it sticking. Add the soy sauce, chilli powder, kidney beans and tomatoes and allow to simmer gently for 20 minutes.

Take the wraps and spread a thin layer of cream cheese in the middle of each. Put about 3 tbsp of the filling on each wrap then sprinkle with grated cheese. Roll the wrap up and serve with some shredded lettuce or salad.

Variations
- You can add a couple of cloves of garlic if you like, plus some red or green chillis.
- Use low-fat plain yoghurt instead of cream cheese.

Recipes to Help You Give Up Sugar

Mexican Chicken (or Quorn) Wraps

This is like the sort of thing you get in your local fast-food chicken joint – but much better (and better for you)! You can buy bags of frozen mixed peppers at the supermarket. These are fine to use instead of fresh, if you prefer.

Serves 2

- 1 medium red onion
- ⅓ of each of a red pepper, a yellow pepper and a green pepper (or one whole pepper)
- 1 medium courgette
- 2 chicken breasts (or 200g Quorn chunks)
- 1 tbsp olive oil
- Soy sauce and Marmite to flavour (1 tsp Marmite in 100ml boiling water)
- 3 corn tortillas or 6 taco shells
- 1 tbsp low-fat soft cheese

Cut the onion in half and slice thinly. Slice the peppers into long thin strips and do the same with the courgette (top and tail it, cut it in two then slice it lengthways to get lots of thin strips). Cut the chicken breasts into cubes and put in a frying pan with the olive oil. As they are cooking, add the sliced vegetables. When they start to sizzle, add the soy sauce plus the boiling water with Marmite. Cook until the chicken is completely done.

Get three wraps and heat them in a microwave for 30 seconds. Take them out and spread a blob of soft cheese over the centre. Take the chicken and vegetable mixture and put some on each of the three wraps. Roll them up, turn the ends over (so you have a 'parcel') and cut in half (can be eaten with your hands but perhaps not a great meal for a first date!). Serve one and a half wraps per person.

Variations
You can customize these wraps in all sorts of ways:
- Grate carrot into them.
- Add chilli and garlic for a 'kick'.
- Use a dollop of yoghurt or low-fat houmous instead of soft cheese.
- Use one of your daily dairy portions by adding low-fat grated cheese such as Edam.
- If you don't want to use cooked vegetables, add shredded lettuce and tomato.
- The chicken wrap is fantastic with fresh coriander.

Recipes to Help You Give Up Sugar

'Quick' Curry

Again, this is one of those recipes you can adapt to suit your taste. Once you've made the following basic recipe, you can either have it as a veggie curry or you can add one of the 'extras' to bulk it out with your protein choice. If you have a bit left over, you can always add a couple of spoonfuls to your jacket potato or heat it up as your breakfast or one of your snacks the next day.

Serves 2
Basic Curry

- 1 medium onion
- 1 green pepper
- 1 tbsp olive oil
- 1 sweet potato, diced
- 1 tsp curry powder (mild, medium or hot, depending on taste)
- 1 clove of garlic, crushed
- 3 tbsp tomato purée
- 300ml water
- ¼ of a cauliflower, chopped

'Extras'

- 2 chicken breasts, diced
- 200g Quorn chunks
- 200g lean ground beef or turkey mince

Dice the onion and chop the pepper into medium-sized pieces (about the size of a stamp) and put in a frying pan with the olive oil. Heat up and cook until the onions are transparent, then add the diced sweet potato and cauliflower. (If you're using chicken, Quorn, beef or turkey, add it at this stage to brown it. Put in some extra oil if needed.) Add the curry powder, crushed garlic and tomato purée and mix in before adding the water to the mixture.

Allow the mixture to simmer for about 15 minutes or until the sweet potatoes and cauliflower are soft. Serve with basmati rice and garnish with some yoghurt mixed with chopped cucumber and mint.

Variation
- If you want a 'creamy' curry, add a couple of tablespoons of plain yoghurt to the mixture once it's off the heat. If you add it while it's cooking it will curdle.

Chicken and Cashew Stir-fry

You may well have had this delicious combination at a Thai or Chinese restaurant. The cashews complement the chicken perfectly, as well as helping to fill you up!

Recipes to Help You Give Up Sugar

Serves 2

Basic Stir-fry

- 2 spring onions, thinly sliced
- 1 onion, chopped
- 1 courgette, sliced into thin strips
- 1 carrot, sliced into thin strips
- 1 tbsp olive or sesame oil
- 150ml water
- 2 tsp soy sauce
- 1 clove of garlic, crushed
- 2cm root ginger (or ginger powder)
- 100g bean sprouts

Chicken and Cashew Ingredients

- 2 chicken breasts, skinned and cubed
- 50g unsalted cashew nuts

Place the spring onions, onion, courgette and carrot in a frying pan or wok with the oil and heat up together. When the vegetables are turning soft and brown, add the chicken, with 2 tbsp of water plus the soy sauce to make it 'sizzle'. Add the garlic, root ginger (grated, using the same grater you'd use for lemon zest) and cashew nuts, as well as the rest of the water, and cook until the chicken is brown and fully cooked. Add the bean sprouts a couple of minutes before the end of cooking time to warm them through. Serve with rice (3 tbsp per person) or Chinese egg thread noodles.

Variations

- Use prawns instead of chicken, or even Quorn or tofu pieces (about 200g).
- Don't be limited by the vegetable ingredients in the list – if there are others you'd like to include (for example, broccoli, cauliflower, cabbage strips or colourful pieces of pepper), go for it.
- Five spice is a fantastic sweet mixture containing star anise and other spices traditionally used in these dishes. You can also add chilli powder or some Tabasco sauce if you want a bit of a 'kick.'

'Meaty' Bolognaise

Most mums have their own version of a Bolognaise. Our favourite is a veggie recipe using Quorn mince – it's a low-fat dish that's had even our meat-hungry husbands fooled! If you want to use meat, turkey mince is a good low-fat alternative to beef. This is a good basic sauce that can be eaten with pasta or a jacket potato. It freezes brilliantly and can be defrosted in the microwave in minutes.

Serves 4

    1 medium onion, finely chopped
    1 tbsp olive oil
    1 red pepper, finely chopped

- 1 small carrot, grated
- 2 cloves of garlic, crushed
- 200g Quorn or turkey mince
- 1 vegetable stock cube (plus 1 tsp Marmite and splash of soy sauce to flavour)
- 1 can of tomatoes (400g)
- Splash of red wine (optional)

Fry the onion in the oil until transparent then add the pepper, carrot and garlic and cook for another minute. Add the Quorn or turkey and brown lightly. Dissolve the stock cube in a pint of boiling water with the Marmite and soy sauce and add half to the mince mixture. Reduce until the mince is browning, then add the tomatoes. Add the wine (if using) then reduce the mixture until thick before adding the rest of the stock mix. Cook for a further 10 minutes before serving.

Variations
- To make a runnier sauce, add a bottle or carton of passata (strained tomatoes).
- Try adding herbs such as oregano and basil for even more flavour.

Quorn Lasagne

Quorn is a delicious alternative to meat. If you want a meat version, use chicken, turkey or even lean beef mince. The basis for it is the Bolognaise sauce, above. This recipe freezes well.

Serves 4

- Bolognaise sauce (see above)
- 1 packet of lasagne sheets

White Sauce

- 30g low-fat margarine (e.g. Olivio or Pure)
- 2 tbsp wholemeal flour
- 600ml skimmed milk (or unsweetened soya milk)
- 120g grated Edam cheese

Make the Bolognaise sauce, as above. Preheat the oven to 375°F/190°C/Gas Mark 5.

To make the white sauce, melt the margarine in a saucepan over a low heat. Remove from the heat and add the flour, mixing to a smooth paste. Gradually add the milk, stirring constantly over a low heat. Bring the contents back to the boil, stirring, before reducing the heat and simmering for 2 minutes. Remove from the heat and add the grated cheese.

Spread some of the Bolognaise sauce (about 1cm) in the bottom of a large lasagne dish. Cover with lasagne sheets, then pour on some of the white sauce followed by another 1cm-deep layer of lasagne. Repeat until you have at least three lasagne layers. Pour white sauce on top, then sprinkle with the grated Edam. Bake for 40 minutes, then grill to get an extra crunchy topping.

Fettucini Carbonara

Serves 2

This great pasta dish can be either veggie or meat-based, depending on your preferences.

    50g button mushrooms, sliced
    100g ham or Quorn 'ham'
    200g cooked fettucini
    30g low-fat margarine (e.g. Olivio or Pure with Sunflower)
    2 tbsp wholemeal flour
    125ml skimmed milk
    30g Edam or low-fat Cheddar cheese
    1 tsp wholegrain mustard
    2 tbsp white wine

Grill the mushrooms until they start releasing their juices. Roughly chop the ham or Quorn 'ham' into small pieces. Cook the pasta as instructed, drain and set aside. Melt the low-fat margarine in a heavy-bottomed saucepan on a medium heat, then remove from the heat. Stir in the flour to make a paste, then put the pan back on a low heat and add the milk a bit at a time, stirring constantly. Turn up the heat until the sauce thickens, then add the cheese, mustard, wine, mushrooms, ham and pasta. Mix thoroughly before serving.

Variation
- Instead of ham or Quorn 'ham', use smoked salmon, chopped into small pieces.

Beef and Lentil Burgers

The lentils give these burgers a great texture and make them a healthier option than normal beefburgers.

Serves 4

    50g dried red or brown lentils
    225g lean minced beef
    1 small onion, grated
    1 tsp Worcestershire or soy sauce
    1 egg
    25g tomato purée
    1 clove of garlic, crushed

Cook the lentils in boiling water for about 20 minutes or until soft. Drain well before adding to the other ingredients. Mix well and add a pinch of salt and pepper to taste. Shape the ingredients into burgers and place on a lightly greased baking tray. Cook at 200°C/400°F/Gas Mark 6 for about 40 minutes or until cooked through, turning halfway to brown both sides. Alternatively, fry over a medium heat until brown and cooked all the way through.

Sweet Potato and Leek Frittata

This recipe is from Dr Sarah Schenker, nutrition scientist at the British Nutrition Foundation.

Serves 2
- 2 sprays of oil
- 250g sweet potato
- 1 clove of garlic, crushed
- 50g leek, sliced
- 1 tsp chopped sage
- 1 egg
- 3 egg whites
- 50ml skimmed milk
- 7g Edam cheese, grated
- Handful of fresh parsley

Preheat the oven to 180°C/350°F/Gas Mark 4. Spray a 25cm round flan dish with the oil. Cut the sweet potato into thin slices and boil until tender.

Heat a non-stick pan, spray with oil and cook the garlic and leek over a low heat until tender. Stir in half the sage. Place half the sweet potato over the base of the prepared flan dish, top with the leek mixture, then the remaining sweet potato. Combine the egg, egg whites, milk, cheese and parsley and pour over the potato, sprinkling with the remaining sage. Bake for 35 minutes.

Feta, Olive and Baby New Potato Salad

This delicious salad gives you all the carbs and protein you need for the perfect light meal.

Serves 2
- 10 baby new potatoes
- 6 cherry tomatoes
- ¼ of a cucumber
- ½ a red onion
- 60g feta cheese
- 2 tbsp black pitted olives, halved

Boil the potatoes until tender. Drain, cut in half and set aside to cool.

Cut the cherry tomatoes in half, dice the cucumber and slice the red onion. Cut the feta cheese into cubes. When the potatoes are cold, add to the rest of the ingredients. Dress with a vinaigrette made up of three parts olive oil to one part vinegar (e.g. 3 tsp olive oil, 1 tsp vinegar).

Recipes to Help You Give Up Sugar

Sausage and Apple Casserole

This dish tastes great with rice or a jacket potato. The apple gives it a lovely sweet/savoury mix – perfect if all you seem to think about is sugar!

Serves 2

- 4 Quorn sausages
- 1 medium red onion
- 1 medium apple
- 1 tbsp olive oil
- 1 tbsp gravy granules
- 1 tsp Marmite
- 285ml boiling water
- 1 can of tomatoes (400g)

Put the sausages in a baking tray and cook in the oven at 200°C/400°F/Gas Mark 6 for 15 minutes (longer if from frozen) or until browned. Remove from the oven and cut into slices about 1cm thick (or bigger, if preferred).

Slice the onion into small pieces and the apple into chunks (slightly smaller than a stock cube). Heat the onion in a frying pan with the olive oil until transparent. Add the sausages and apple and fry together. Dissolve the gravy granules and Marmite in the water, pour into the frying pan and simmer together on a low heat for 5 minutes. Add the tomatoes and simmer for another 10 minutes. Serve with jacket potatoes or rice.

Variation
- Add a handful of sultanas during cooking for an even more sweet and savoury taste.

Herby Cod Fillets

Serves 2

    2 cod fillets (around 100g each)
    10g wholemeal breadcrumbs
    1 tsp chopped dill
    1 tsp chopped parsley
    1 tsp chopped chives
    1 tsp low-fat fromage frais
    5 cherry tomatoes, quartered
    1 tsp lemon juice
    Freshly ground pepper

Preheat the oven to 180°C/350°F/Gas Mark 4.

Season the cod fillets and place in a foil-lined roasting tin, skin side down.

In a bowl mix together the other ingredients and spoon some on top of each fillet, packing down gently. Cook for 20 minutes.

Recipes to Help You Give Up Sugar

Tuna Macaroni Bake

Serves 2

- 200g macaroni pasta
- 1 onion, chopped
- 1 clove of garlic
- 1 tbsp olive oil
- 1 medium courgette, grated
- 1 can of tomatoes (400g)
- 1 small can of sweetcorn
- 1 can of tuna (200g), drained
- 125g cottage cheese
- 50g 'grainy' breadcrumbs
- 60g grated Edam

Preheat the oven to 180°C/350°F/Gas Mark 4.

Cook the pasta for half the time specified on the pack – about 5 minutes. Drain and set aside.

Fry the onion, garlic and grated courgette together in the oil until they start to brown. Stir in the tomatoes and sweetcorn and heat through. Add to the pasta along with the tuna and cottage cheese. Stir well before placing in an ovenproof dish. Top with breadcrumbs and the grated Edam. Bake for about 30 minutes until the top has browned. Serve with salad and/or vegetables.

Variation

You can use chicken, Quorn or turkey instead of tuna.

SIDE DISHES

Potato Wedges

Once you've made your own potato wedges, you'll never bother buying frozen ones from the supermarket again (especially as you now know they may have sugar lurking in them). Like the shop-bought ones, our wedges include the skins. But we use sweet potatoes as well as conventional potatoes because they have a great, sweet taste and a low GI (see page 41).

Serves 2
- 100g potato
- 100g sweet potato
- ½ tsp soy sauce
- ½ tsp ground chilli powder
- 1 tsp olive oil

Preheat the oven to 375°F/190°C/Gas Mark 5.

Scrub the potato and sweet potato then chop into wedges (about the same size as orange segments), leaving the skins on. Mix the soy sauce and chilli powder in with the olive oil. Put the oil mix in a baking tray with the wedges. Mix them up so that the wedges are covered with the oil mix on all sides. Bake for 25 minutes, turning after 15 minutes. They should be well browned when you remove them. If you want them extra brown, put the baking tray on the hob and brown for a further five minutes, turning so that they don't burn.

Ratatouille

This is packed full of vegetable goodness and is easy to make – just chop, chuck in a pan and leave to cook.

Serves 2

- 1 tsp olive oil
- ½ a courgette, sliced
- ½ a carrot, sliced
- ½ an aubergine, diced
- 1 small onion, diced
- 450g mushrooms, sliced or quartered
- 1 tin chopped tomatoes (400g)
- 1 tbsp tomato purée
- 1 clove of garlic, crushed
- 1 tsp oregano

Heat the olive oil in a pan, add the onion and cook until transparent. Add the other vegetables and cook together for a couple of minutes before adding the tomatoes, tomato purée, garlic and oregano. Cook for about 30 minutes until thickened (add a little water if you want it 'sloppier'). Serve with basmati rice or a baked potato, or with some chicken breasts.

Spicy Noodles

These tasty noodles are a great accompaniment to fish cakes or a simple fish steak such as tuna.

Serves 2

- 150g egg noodles
- 2 tsp olive or sesame oil
- 1 tsp sesame seeds
- ½ a red onion, finely chopped
- 6 baby sweetcorn
- 12 mangetout pods
- 1 red pepper, cut into strips
- 1 spring onion, finely sliced
- 2cm piece of fresh ginger, peeled and grated
- 1 fresh red chilli, finely sliced
- Chilli or Tabasco sauce
- 1 tsp soy sauce

Prepare the noodles according to the instructions on the packet. Drain and set aside.

Heat the oil in a frying pan and add the sesame seeds, onion and vegetables, stir-frying for 2 minutes. Stir in the ginger and red chilli and fry for another couple of minutes. Add the drained noodles to the mixture and stir-fry for a minute before adding the chilli and soy sauces.

Variations
- Add as many different kinds of vegetables as you like, including courgettes, peas or cabbage.
- Try adding a few nuts.

Carrot and Sultana Salad

This lovely light salad goes perfectly with grilled meat or fish dishes.

Serves 2

150g carrots, grated
50g sultanas
1 tsp toasted sesame seeds
½ tsp balsamic vinegar
1½ tsp olive oil

Grate the carrots into a bowl and mix in the sultanas and sesame seeds. Add the vinegar and olive oil and mix well.

Variation

Try chopping other vegetables into the salad too, such as spring onions or baby sweetcorn.

Sweet Pasta Salad

This easy salad is great with a protein such as chicken, a fish fillet, a lean chop or some fish cakes. The apple and beetroot give the dish a great sweetness and a beautiful colour!

Serves 2

- 200g pasta (e.g. bows or shells)
- 1 tsp olive oil
- 1 tsp cider vinegar
- 1 tsp Dijon mustard
- 1 clove of garlic, crushed
- Ground black pepper, to taste
- 1 apple, diced
- 1 cooked beetroot, diced

Cook the pasta following the packet instructions or until 'al dente'.

Mix together the oil, vinegar, mustard, garlic and pepper. Chop the apple and beetroot and mix in with the pasta and the dressing. Serve chilled.

Variations
- For extra sweetness, add some chopped apricots or sultanas.
- Try adding a few walnuts.

Healthier 'Mayo'

Even some 'light' shop-bought mayonnaises contain sugar, so here's a sugar-free version you can use in recipes or as part of a sandwich filling. For each sandwich, use 1 tbsp of 'mayo'.

> 2 tbsp quark or low-fat fromage frais
> 1 tbsp low-fat yoghurt
> Salt and freshly ground black pepper
> Squeeze of lemon or lime juice

Mix the quark and yoghurt together before adding the salt, pepper and juice. Keep in a container in the fridge and stir before use.

Variations
- Add some paprika or even some chilli for a different flavour.
- Use a light cream cheese instead of the quark or fromage frais.

DESSERTS

Bread and Butter Pudding

We've modified this old favourite by making it without sugar. But the dried fruit gives it plenty of sweetness so you shouldn't feel you're missing out.

Serves 2
- 4 slices of wholemeal bread, crusts removed
- 1 tsp butter or margarine
- 25g seedless raisins
- 300ml skimmed milk
- 1 large egg, beaten
- Grated rind of ½ an orange
- ½ tsp ground cinnamon

Grease an oven-proof dish. Spread the bread with the butter or margarine and cut into strips. Place a layer of bread in the base of the dish, butter side up. Sprinkle with raisins and cover with more bread and raisins to create layers.

Warm the milk in a saucepan and stir in the egg, orange rind and cinnamon. Pour over the bread and allow to stand for around 15 minutes. Cook at 170°C/325°F/Gas Mark 3 for 45 minutes until the top is golden brown. Serve with fresh yoghurt, fromage frais or sugarless custard.

Variations
- Grate some fresh nutmeg on top.
- Use mixed dried fruit instead of (or as well as) the raisins.

Custard

This is like custard but without all that sugar. Eat it with Fruit Mix (page 298), Bread and Butter Pudding (above) or simply a chopped banana – delicious!

Serves 2
1 tbsp fine maize meal or cornflour
400ml semi-skimmed milk
1 large egg
1 tsp vanilla essence
Grated nutmeg

Put the fine maize meal in a mixing bowl and add enough milk to make a paste. Add the egg and mix together. Heat the rest of the milk in a saucepan before stirring in the paste. Cook on a low heat, stirring constantly, while the custard thickens. Stir for another couple of minutes before adding the vanilla essence. Sprinkle with grated nutmeg to serve.

SUGAR ADDICTS' DIET

Vanilla and Strawberry Tofu Ice Cream

If you love ice cream but can't justify the sugar content, make your own. This version uses tofu (made from soya beans, a great form of low-fat protein) and low-fat yoghurt, as well as plenty of fruit. The vanilla essence gives it a lovely flavour reminiscent of 'real' ice cream.

Serves 2
- 3 tbsp silken tofu
- 3 tbsp plain yoghurt
- 200g mango (fresh or tinned)
- 2 tbsp vanilla essence
- 200g strawberries

Mix the tofu, yoghurt and mango together in a blender. Add vanilla essence to taste – put in more if you want a stronger flavour. Chop the strawberries into quarters or slice them and add to the mixture (don't liquidize). Pour into a plastic container with a lid (such as an empty ice-cream tub) and freeze. Remove from the freezer half an hour before serving to soften.

Variations
- The possibilities are endless! Try using any fruit that takes your fancy, such as blackberries, raspberries, bananas, papaya, pears or peaches. Use fresh or even tinned fruit (in its own juice, not syrup).

- Try using other flavourings instead of the vanilla, such as almond essence, cinnamon, dried coconut or even sugar-free carob for a chocolate-style ice cream.
- If you don't want to use tofu, use more plain yoghurt instead.

Lemon Cheesecake

For the base:
   8 rye crispbreads (e.g. Ryvita)
   1 tbsp butter

For the topping:
   Cottage cheese
   Grated rind and juice of half a lemon
   1 tsp vanilla essence
   Cinammon (optional)

Crush the rye crispbreads in a blender or put in a sandwich bag and bash with a rolling pin or can. Add the butter and mix well until you have a firm ball of mixture. Press the base mixture into a cake tin and put in the fridge to cool for a couple of hours.

Liquidize the cottage cheese until smooth before adding a squeeze of lemon juice (about 1 tsp) plus the grated rind and vanilla essence. Spoon the mixture on top of the base. Sprinkle on some more rind plus some cinnamon (optional) for extra flavour and decoration.

Chill for another hour before serving.

Variations
- For a different topping flavour, use orange or lime juice instead of lemon juice.
- Add some ground cinnamon to the base mix for a different taste.

Pancakes

This versatile recipe can be used with both sweet and savoury toppings. We love it with puréed banana and cinnamon but try it with chopped fresh fruit, cottage cheese or low-fat cheese. Experiment – the possibilities are endless. You can make a batch of pancakes in advance – put them in the fridge covered with a damp cloth (e.g. a tea towel) to keep them moist, then heat them up in a microwave or conventional oven.

Makes about 12 pancakes
    125g wholemeal flour
    1 large egg
    350ml semi-skimmed milk
    1 tbsp oil
    A pinch of salt
    Knob of butter (or olive oil) for cooking

Put the sieved flour into a mixing bowl and make a hole in the centre. Break in the egg and mix together with a fork. Pour the milk in a little at a time, and whisk the mixture until thickened, like cream.

Heat a frying pan then add the butter (or oil). Drop in 2 tbsp of the mix and cook until set before turning it over and cooking the other side. Serve with whatever mixture you want.

Variation

Put some flavouring in the pancake mix, such as cinnamon or vanilla.

SNACKS

Tuna Pâté

Serves 2 (or makes 2 snack portions)
- 1 small tin tuna
- 125g cottage cheese
- 2 drops lemon juice
- Black pepper

Drain any liquid from the tuna before putting it in a liquidizer (if it's too 'wet' the pâté will be runny). Add the cottage cheese and lemon juice and liquidize until smooth. Season with pepper to taste. Put in a storage box in the fridge and use on bread, rice cakes, in wholemeal pitta bread or rye crispbreads.

Variations
- For a different flavoured pâté, replace the tuna with chopped chicken or turkey breast or smoked mackerel.
- Add herbs to make it more interesting – try dill with the fish versions and parsley with the meat ones.

Celery Cheese Fillers

Serves 1

   1 tsp sesame seeds
   Low-fat soft cheese (e.g. Philadelphia Light)
   4 sticks of celery

Mix the sesame seeds with the soft cheese. Spread it into the celery sticks and cut into small pieces to eat.

Variations
- Use cottage cheese instead of cream cheese, either plain or a flavoured (but not sugared!) version such as onion and chive.
- Try other seeds such as sunflower or pumpkin.
- Use red, yellow or orange peppers instead of celery.

Recipes to Help You Give Up Sugar

Tortilla Chips and Salsa

If you love 'chips and dips', this is a recipe for you. Shop-bought dips – or 'salsas' – tend to be loaded with sugar. Choose plain or lightly salted tortilla chips rather than flavoured ones, which often contain lots of additives and even sugar. This salsa also tastes great with rye crispbread – spread with a thin layer of cream cheese then top with the salsa. Delicious!

Serves 2
- ½ an onion, chopped
- 1 clove of garlic, crushed
- 1 can of chopped tomatoes (400g)
- 1 red chilli, finely chopped
- Fresh coriander

Fry the onion and garlic until brown then add the chopped tomatoes and chilli. Simmer for about 10 minutes. Finely chop the fresh coriander and add to the mixture. Take off the heat and leave to cool. Serve with tortilla chips and some low-fat cheese or yoghurt for a good carb/protein snack.

Afterword: What Next

If you've been following the Sugar Addicts' Diet plan, you should be starting to settle into this new way of exercising, eating and thinking about food. Even if you've just read the book and haven't yet started on the plan, the information you've picked up has probably made you something of an expert when it comes to spotting sugars!

So what next? We'll be overjoyed if you end up feeling like Nicki has as a result of devising this diet plan and sticking to it – happier, free from cravings and, yes, a few pounds lighter. We know it's possible because it happened to her. Remember, although she felt better within three weeks, for some people it can take up to six weeks.

The next stage for you is to carry on using the plan and seeing it as a way of life rather than a diet. And once you've done this, your diet should be so healthy and balanced that you can incorporate a little sugar or foods with artificial sweeteners into your diet. But if you're like Nicki, you'll find your cravings have subsided anyway, so sweet foods may not be as alluring as they once were. Nicki would once have walked over hot coals to get to sweets but now she can take them or leave them. Yes, really!

SUGAR ADDICTS' DIET

In the meantime, we'd like to say, 'Keep up the good work.' Kicking out those extra sugars can really make a difference to your quality of life, as well as helping you secure a healthier future. **Being free from sugar addiction could be the best thing that's ever happened to you.**

Bibliography

Andrews, Dr S. *et al. Sugar Busters!*, Random House, 1998
Barnard, N. *Breaking the Food Seduction*, St Martin's Press, 2003
Brand-Miller *et al. The New Glucose Revolution*, Marlowe & Company, 2003
Budd, M. & M. *Eat to Beat Low Blood Sugar*, Thorsons, 2003
Critser, G. *Fat Land*, Penguin, 2004
DesMaisons, K. *The Sugar Addict's Total Recovery Programme*, Simon & Schuster, 2000
Erasmus, U. *Fats that Heal Fats that Kill,* Alive Books, 1993
Geary, A. *The Food and Mood Handbook*, Thorsons, 2004
Haynes, A.J. *The Insulin Factor*, Thorsons, 2004
Lefever, Dr R. *Break Free from Addiction*, Carlton, 2003
McCance and Widdowson. *The Composition of Foods*, The Royal Society of Chemistry and The Food Standards Agency, 2002
Murray, M. *Encyclopedia of Nutritional Supplements*, Prima, 1996
Nestlé, M. *Food Politics: How the Food Industry*

Influences Nutrition and Health, University of California Press, 2003
Ursell A. *'L' is for Labels*, Hay House, 2004
Vale, J. *Chocolate Busters: The Easy Way to Kick It!*, Thorsons, 2004
White, E. *Beat Candida Cookbook*, Thorsons, 1999
Young, W. *Sold Out: The True Cost of Supermarket Shopping*, Vision Paperbacks, 2004

Useful Organizations

FOOD

British Nutrition Foundation
For information on food and nutritional requirements.
www.nutrition.org.uk

British Association for Nutritional Therapy
For information on how to find a nutritional therapist
www.bant.org.uk

British Dietetic Association
For information on how to find a dietician.
www.bda.uk.com

The Parents Jury
An independent jury of parents which seeks to improve the quality of children's foods and drinks.
www.parentsjury.org

The Food Commission
Independent pressure group campaigning for safer food.
www.foodcomm.org.uk

The Food Standards Agency
The government's food watchdog.
www.foodstandards.gov.uk

Sustain
Independent pressure group campaigning for better food and agricultural policies.
www.sustain.org

Consumers' Association
Campaigning for the rights of UK consumers.
www.which.net

Health
British Heart Foundation
Heart health information charity.
www.bhf.org.uk

Diabetes UK
Diabetes help and information charity.
www.diabetes.org.uk

Cancer Research UK
Visit the charity's special CancerHelp UK website for advice and information.
www.cancerhelp.org.uk

Useful Organizations

Weight Concern
A registered charity committed to addressing the physical and psychological health needs of overweight and obese people.
www.weightconcern.com

National Obesity Forum
Organization aiming to raise awareness of the impact of obesity.
www.nationalobesityforum.org.uk

Sport England
Find out more about getting into sports and exercise.
www.sportengland.org